EAT
RIGHT
FOR
YOUR
SIGHT

THE EXPERIMENT

BECAUSE EVERY BOOK IS A TEST OF NEW IDEAS

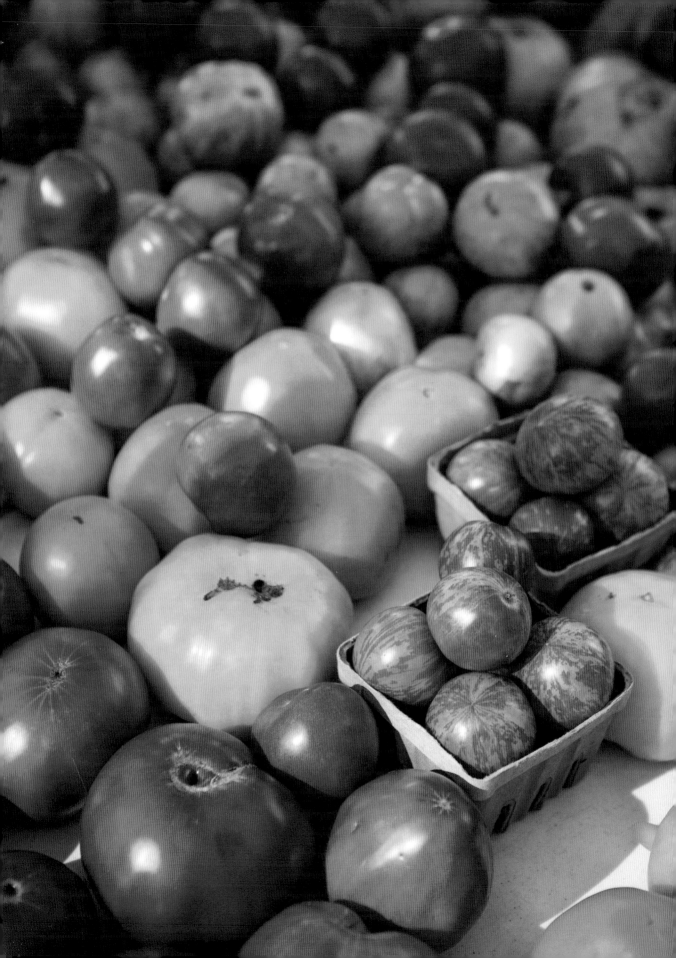

Jennifer Trainer Thompson
Johanna M. Seddon, MD, ScM

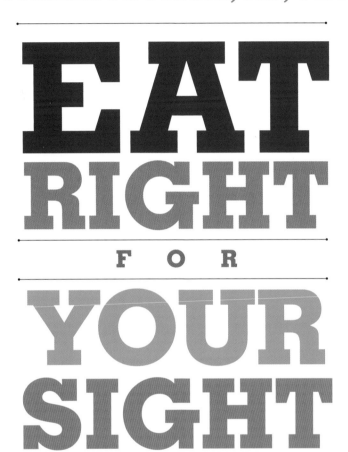

EAT RIGHT FOR YOUR SIGHT

Simple, Tasty Recipes That Help Reduce
the Risk of Vision Loss from Macular Degeneration

A PROJECT OF THE
American Macular Degeneration Foundation

THE EXPERIMENT

NEW YORK

The Experiment, LLC
220 East 23rd Street, Suite 301
New York, NY 10010-4674
www.theexperimentpublishing.com

This book contains the opinions and ideas of its authors. It is intended to provide helpful and informative material on the subjects addressed in the book. It is sold with the understanding that the authors and publisher are not engaged in rendering medical, health, or any other kind of personal professional services in the book. The authors and publisher specifically disclaim all responsibility for any liability, loss, or risk—personal or otherwise—that is incurred as a consequence, directly or indirectly, of the use and application of any of the contents of this book.

The Experiment's books are available at special discounts when purchased in bulk for premiums and sales promotions as well as for fund-raising or educational use. For details, contact us at info@theexperimentpublishing.com.

Library of Congress Cataloging-in-Publication Data

Thompson, Jennifer Trainer.
  Eat right for your sight : simple, tasty recipes that help reduce the risk of vision loss from macular degeneration / Jennifer Trainer Thompson, Johanna M. Seddon, MD, ScM.
      pages cm
  Includes index.
  "First published in slightly different form as a hardcover in 2014 as Feast for the Eyes® by American Macular Degeneration Foundation"--Preliminaries.
  ISBN 978-1-61519-249-6 (pbk.) -- ISBN 978-1-61519-250-2 (ebook) 1. Retinal degeneration--Diet therapy--Recipes. 2. Retinal degeneration--Prevention. I. Seddon, Johanna M. II. American Macular Degeneration Foundation. III. Title.
  RE661.D3T46 2015
  641.5'63--dc23
                                          2014036057

ISBN 978-1-61519-249-6
Ebook ISBN 978-1-61519-250-2

Additional photographs by Paul Rocheleau
Food Styling by Catrine Kelty
Chip Goehring, Editorial Director
Rosalind Torrey, Editorial Supervisor
Karen J. Westergaard, Editorial Assistant
Paul F. Gariepy, Chief Proofreader
Mark Torrey, Online Consultant
Michael Trotman, Copyeditor
The Lisa Ekus Group, LLC, Editorial Consultants
Cover design by Susi Oberhelman
Cover photographs by Jason Houston
Original text design by Hans Teensma, Impress
Text design and typesetting by Pauline Neuwirth, Neuwirth & Associates, Inc.

Manufactured in China
Distributed by Workman Publishing Company, Inc.
Distributed simultaneously in Canada by Thomas Allen & Son Ltd.

First printing February 2015
10 9 8 7 6 5 4 3 2 1

Contents

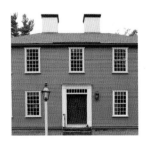
Small Bites

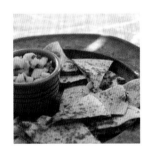

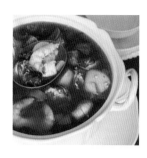

Soups

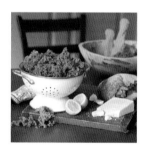

Salads

Main Courses

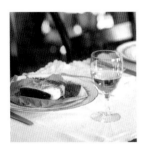

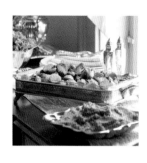

Side Dishes

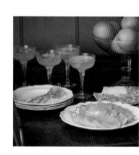

Desserts

Healthy Drinks

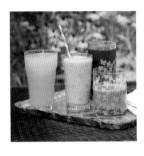

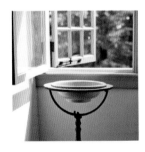

Foreword

It's not all carrots and spinach

This book will give you some deliciously memorable meals and it may also help save your eyesight. Not bad for a modest investment.

Indulge me for a moment in a back story. Months after my 39th birthday, my ophthalmologist told me I might go blind from an eye disease I had never heard of and could barely pronounce: macular degeneration. For a while I called it "molecular degeneration." This was in early 1993, pre–World Wide Web, and at the time most doctors thought there was little, if anything, that could be done to stop the disease's progression. I was shocked and confused. Like most people, I'd heard of cataracts and glaucoma, but I had never heard of macular degeneration. Why was that? And where was the information I needed to find out more about my condition?

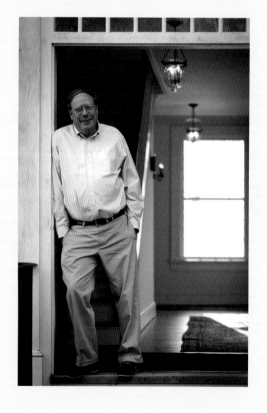

I quit practicing law, started talking to researchers who knew a lot about macular degeneration and, with the help of many, founded the American Macular Degeneration Foundation. I couldn't prevent others from getting the same bad news I had received, but I could at least provide the information, support, and resources to do something about the situation.

As I came to learn, macular degeneration affects central vision and is the leading cause of legal blindness in people over 55 years old in the Western world. In the United States alone, it affects ten million people, some in midlife like me, and the number is expected to grow as baby boomers age. What it is not, however, is a sure sentence of blindness. Twenty years after my diagnosis, I can still see and read, though with a bit of difficulty. I drive, even at night, work, and function well. Do I consider myself lucky? Certainly: I feel fortunate that 20 years ago, some researchers shared with me the names of foods and supplements they believed might help slow the progress of my disease.

Two decades of ongoing research have proven the scientists right. This issue is so important to me that I opened up my home in rural western Massachusetts to a talented team of food professionals and over the course of many months we created this book. All these meals were created in my kitchen at my table from seasonal ingredients. This cookbook is a way to incorporate the science behind vision health and overall well-being into daily life. The recipes are easy to live with and tasty to boot. Red curry vegetables, grilled salmon—these are not exactly deprivation foods, and they're good for the eyes. I'm glad to know that my runny, gooey, yolky eggs also benefit my vision. I love corn, blueberries, strawberries, and sweet red peppers anyway, and now that I know they're medicine for what ails me, I eat them more often. You owe it to yourself to dig in. With the help of such diverse recipes in this book, I don't get tired of the foods I need most. Admittedly, the mighty kale has been more of an acquired taste, but it can be prepared to suit your palate. Everyone can benefit, even if your eyes are just fine.

I am grateful to those doctors who spend their professional lives searching for prevention and treatment for macular degeneration. Now there is a book that takes some of that knowledge and puts it in our own hands. So get reacquainted with your produce aisle and your local farmers market. Shop and cook from the recipes in this book. Eat and enjoy. These recipes are, literally, a feast for the eyes.

Chip Goehring
President, Board of Trustees
American Macular Degeneration Foundation

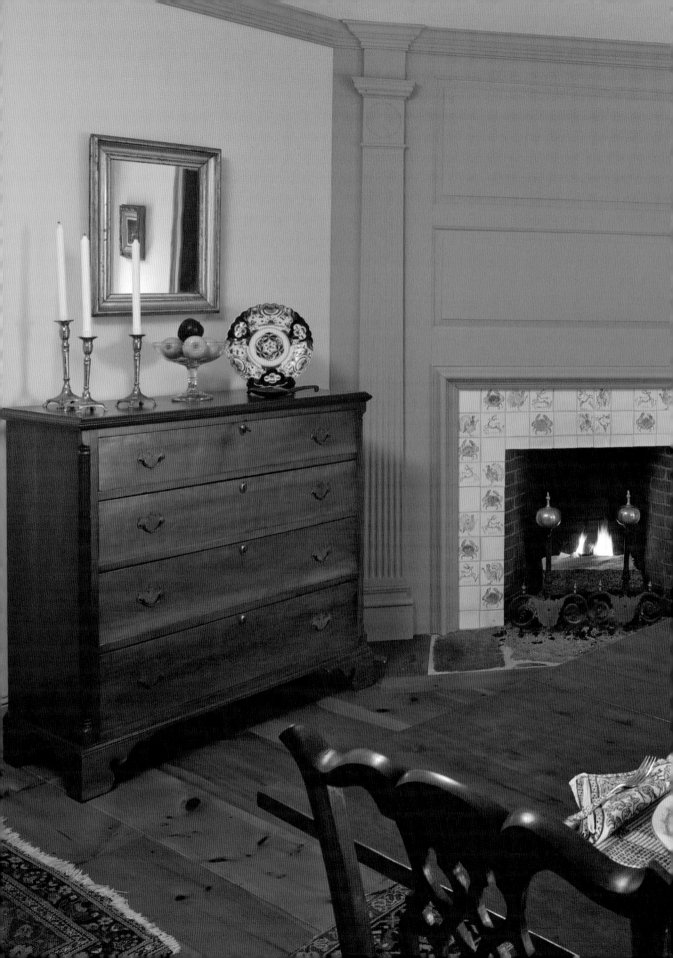

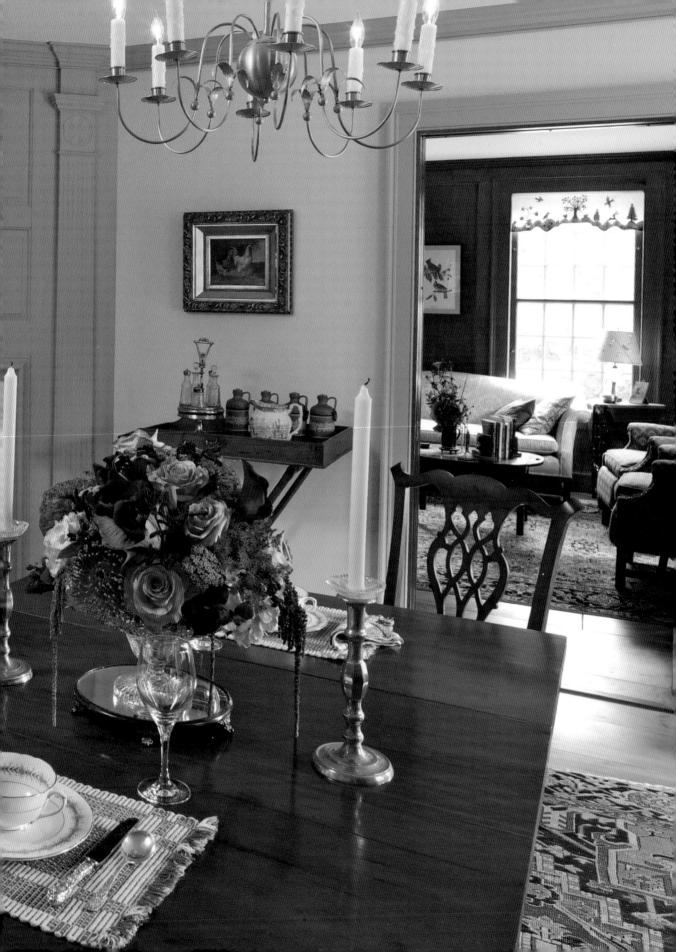

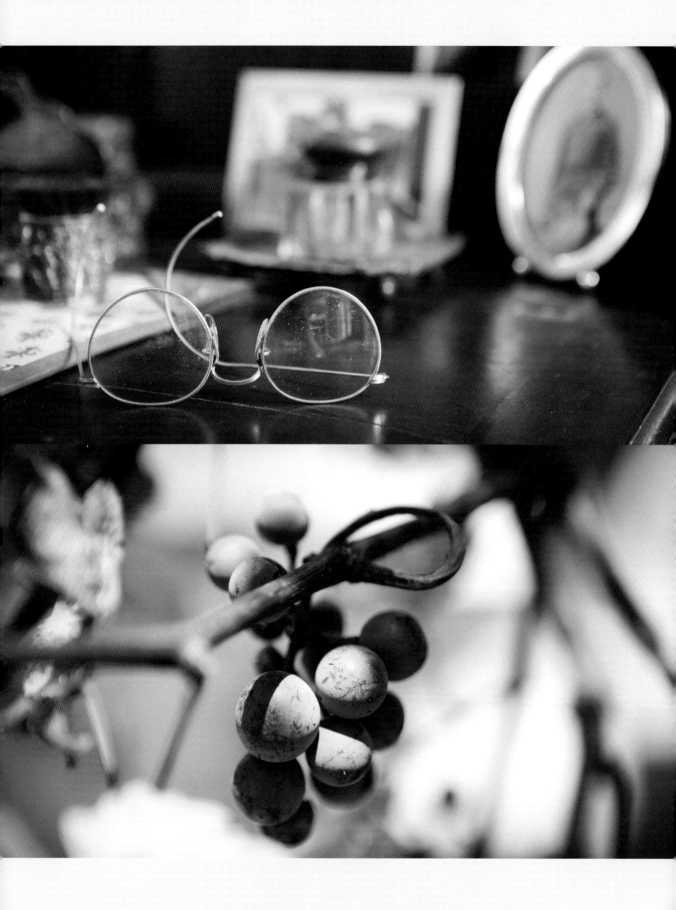

What Is Age-Related Macular Degeneration (AMD)?

Age-related macular degeneration (AMD) is damage to or breakdown of the central part of the retina, called the macula, which allows us to see details clearly. Macular degeneration can impair both distance and close vision, but does not affect peripheral (side) vision. Macular degeneration by itself does not cause total blindness, but can result in complete loss of central vision.

There are two types of macular degeneration: dry and wet. "Dry" (atrophic) macular degeneration is the result of drusen (protein and lipid deposits) forming in the macula and is the more common form of the disease. Vision loss is gradual. The most advanced form of the dry type is called geographic atrophy. "Wet" (exudative) macular degeneration occurs when abnormal blood vessels form underneath the retina and leak fluid or blood. This type accounts for about 10 percent of macular degeneration, and vision loss can be rapid and severe.

Many people, including Georgia O'Keeffe, Judi Dench, and Stephen King have experienced the telltale sign of seeing an area of darkness in the middle of their vision, making even the simplest tasks—driving, reading, recognizing faces—difficult to impossible. Although the disease can strike patients of any age (a rare form of the disease affects children), macular degeneration is often related to aging, and the percentage of the American population over 65 is increasing rapidly. Experts predict the elderly population will be six times greater in 2025 than in 1990; thus the disease is likely to approach epidemic proportions.

Healthy Foods for Your Eyes

"Tell me what you eat, and I will tell you what you are."
— *Brillat-Savarin*

Certain nutrients are vital to eye growth and development. They are obtained in one of two ways: as vitamin A, in sources such as liver, fish oils, egg yolks, and dairy products, and as a precursor to vitamin A, called carotenoids (such as beta-carotene or alpha-carotene), which are found in and lend the pigment to colorful fruits and vegetables like carrots, squash, broccoli, sweet potatoes, apricots, and leafy greens. The body converts the carotenoids to retinol (a type of vitamin A) in the small intestine. Other carotenoids are lutein and zeaxanthin, pigments that give certain plants their characteristic color. High concentrations of lutein and zeaxanthin are found in dark green vegetables, especially spinach, kale, turnip greens, collard greens, romaine lettuce, squash, broccoli, peas, and brussels sprouts; orange and yellow fruits and vegetables including oranges, papayas, tangerines, peaches, corn, tomatoes, pumpkins, and carrots; and even egg yolks. Parsley also has some of these nutrients.

Lutein and zeaxanthin are antioxidants that are found naturally in the macula (the center of the retina) and need to be replenished regularly. There is some evidence that consuming a diet rich in carotenoids may reduce the risk of developing age-related macular degeneration (AMD).

Another class of nutrients is polyphenols, a large class of chemical compounds synthesized by fruits, vegetables, and beverages such as juices and teas that have antioxidant, anti-inflammatory, and anticarcinogenic properties. The major sources of polyphenols in the average diet are flavonoids, which may help blood flow to the retina while fighting free-radical damage from ultraviolet sunrays. Flavonoids are plentiful in broccoli, blueberries, limes, oranges, lemons, onions,

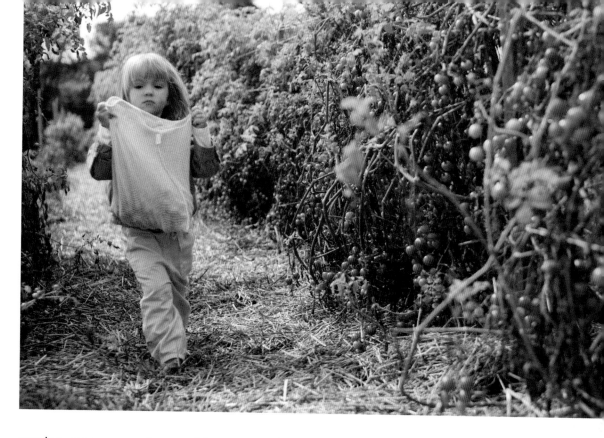

apples, pomegranates, and tomatoes. Another polyphenol is catechin—green tea in particular is made from unfermented tea leaves and reportedly contains the highest concentration of catechins in any food. While tea leaves are a good source of catechins, they can also be found in cocoa, acai oil, peaches, and vinegar.

Other foods to look for:

- Foods containing selenium, a trace mineral absorbed into proteins, help protect cells from damage caused by free radicals. Selenium is found in brown rice, wheat, eggs, tuna, shrimp, sunflower seeds, Brazil nuts, and chicken.

- Foods strong in vitamin D3, such as fortified milk, salmon, mackerel, sardines, egg yolks, and beef liver, help the body absorb calcium and, along with calcium, help protect against osteoporosis.

- Foods rich in vitamin C, a powerful antioxidant, can protect against free radicals, which are thought to contribute to AMD. Examples include red and green bell peppers, fruits, cauliflower, and green cabbage.

- Foods rich in vitamin E (which is a powerful antioxidant, and important for a healthy immune system, skin, and eyes) include broccoli, peanuts, almonds, avocados, mangoes, and sunflower seeds.

- Omega-3 fatty acids, which support the healthy development of the brain, nerves, and eyes, and are plentiful in fish (salmon, sardines, herring, mackerel, and other fatty fish, and in smaller amounts in halibut, cod, shrimp, and scallops). Other forms can be found in flaxseeds, walnuts, squash, tofu, and soybeans.

- Zinc contributes to a strong immune system, helps your skin stay healthy, and heals wounds. Recent studies suggest zinc can also slow progression of macular degeneration. Sources include meat, seafood (especially oysters and crab), nuts, and whole grains.

- Anthocyanin is a fancy name for certain purple, blue, or red antioxidants that may help bolster collagen structure in the retina. You'll find them in grapes, blueberries, pomegranates, cranberries, and other dark foods.

- Lycopene, part of the carotenoid family, occurs naturally in fruits and vegetables such as tomatoes. (It is the pigment that makes tomatoes red. The redder the tomato, the more lycopene is present.) Other good sources include pink grapefruit, watermelon, and papaya.

If you are sodium sensitive, consider using salt alternatives.

Vitamin A supplements are recommended for patients with retinitis pigmentosa, but patients with Stargardt disease should not *take vitamin A supplements.*

Visit macular.org for updates and further nutritional information.

> "We are indeed much more than what we eat, but what we eat can nevertheless help us to be much more than what we are." — *Adelle Davis*

Proper nutrition is critical to eye health, and it's important to know not only what to eat, but also how much. While it's always best to get essential vitamins and minerals from foods, some of the recommended amounts below may be difficult to achieve without taking supplements. Talk to your doctor or registered dietitian, using this list as a starting point to getting the right amounts of eye-healthy nutrients.

Nutrient	Found in	USDA Dietary Reference Intake	RDA for Ocular Health
Beta-carotene*	Carrots, spinach, cantaloupe, pumpkins, turnip greens, winter squash, cabbage	No recommended amount	15,000 µg (15 mg)
Lutein / Zeaxanthin	Kale, spinach, collard greens, turnip greens, corn, green peas, broccoli, tomatoes, eggs	No recommended amount	6,000–10,000 µg / 2,000 µg (6–10 mg / 2 mg)
Omega-3 Fatty Acids	Salmon, walnuts, canola oil, flaxseeds, sardines, mackerel	No recommended amount	1 g (1,000 mg)
Vitamin A	Sweet potatoes, carrots, beef liver, fortified milk, dried herbs, butternut squash, dried apricots	2,300 IU (women) 3,000 IU (men)	Varies
Vitamin C	Oranges, kiwi, red peppers, grapefruit juice, straw-berries, papayas	75–90 mg	500 mg
Vitamin D**	Fortified milk, cod liver oil, salmon, herring, mushrooms, beef liver, eggs	600 IU (adults 19–70) 800 IU (71 and older)	1,000–2,000 IU
Vitamin E	Salad dressing, oils, almonds, sunflower seeds, wheat germ, peanut butter, avocados	22 IU	200–400 IU
Zinc	Fortified breakfast cereal, shellfish, beef, cocoa powder, peanuts	8–11 mg	20–80 mg

Source: USDA and ocular nutrition research literature.

* Current or past smokers should avoid taking nutritional supplements with beta-carotene.

** Based on observational studies of eye disease.

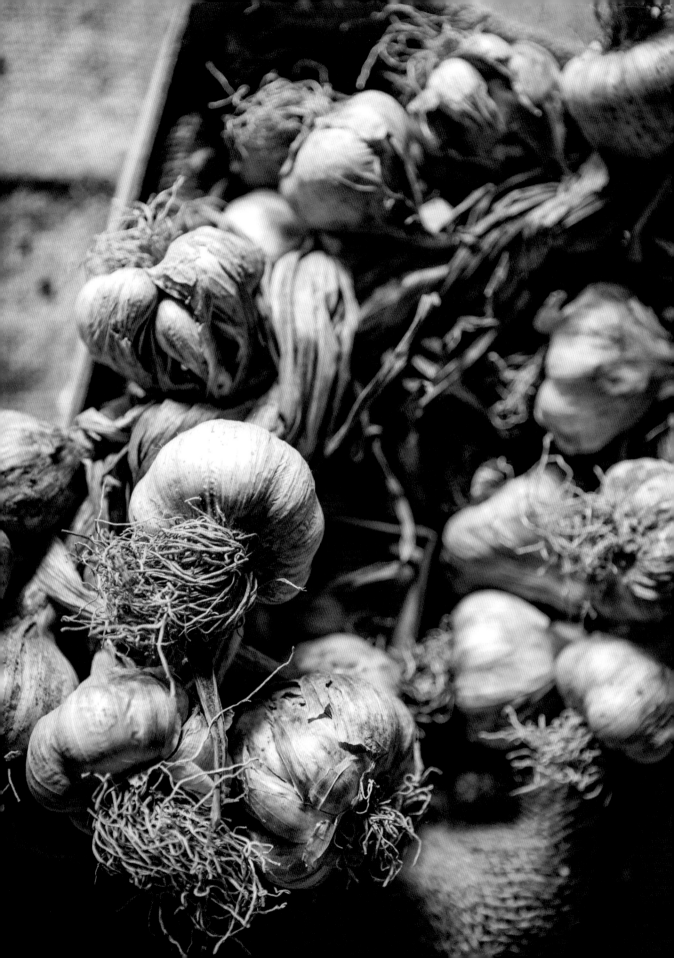

Foods to Have in Your Pantry

FRUIT *(fresh or frozen)*
Apples
Avocados
Blackberries
Blueberries
Cantaloupe
Cranberries
Dried fruits
Grapefruit
Kiwi
Lemons
Oranges
Peaches
Raspberries
Strawberries

SEEDS AND NUTS
Almonds
Flaxseeds
Peanut butter
Sunflower seeds
Walnuts

GRAINS AND PASTAS
Brown rice
Couscous
Pasta
Quinoa
Whole grain bread

VEGETABLES
Broccoli
Cabbage
Carrots
Corn
Garlic
Green peas
Greens (e.g., kale, spinach)
Onions
Peppers
Squash
Sweet potatoes
Tomatoes *(fresh or canned, no salt)*

BEANS AND SOY
Chickpeas
Dried and canned beans
Edamame (soybeans)
Lentils
Tofu

OILS
Canola oil
Flaxseed oil
Olive oil

DAIRY
Cheese *(low-fat or skim)*
Eggs
Milk *(low-fat or skim)*
Plain yogurt *(low-fat or fat-free)*

MEATS/SEAFOOD
Chicken
Herring
Lean beef
Lean pork
Mackerel
Oysters
Salmon *(fresh or canned)*
Sardines
Scallops
Shrimp
Tuna
Turkey

Introduction

You Are What You Eat by Victor Lindlahr was a book that my father had in our home when I was growing up in Pittsburgh in the 1950s and early '60s. My father, a coal-mining son of a coal miner, became a champion of holistic health and natural medicine in an era when canned, processed, and pesticide-laden foods held glittery state-of-the-art appeal. His formal education had ended at age 12, but by the time he turned 40 he had self-educated his way out of the mines to become the local secretary-treasurer of the United Mine Workers of America. From this vantage point he saw tragic consequences of unsafe work conditions and unhealthy lifestyles. He and my mother taught me and our family that the adage "you are what you eat" was plain and obvious truth.

Years later, in medical school at the University of Pittsburgh, I distinctly remember my father showing me a news article concerning a Canadian doctor who was testing vitamin E as a treatment for an eye problem related to prematurity in babies (retinopathy of prematurity). My father's inspiration and my own curiosity soon led me to study the relationships among nutrition, antioxidants, and eye diseases, including macular degeneration, long before these connections became accepted.

After medical school, I completed my ophthalmology residency at Tufts New England Medical Center and became the first ophthalmologist to have obtained a graduate degree in epidemiology at the Harvard School of Public Health. This education and preparation enabled me to found a research division at Harvard to study the prevention of eye diseases and initiate nutritional studies of macular degeneration and cataracts.

When I began my career as an ophthalmologist and retina specialist, a large percentage of my patients were elderly with macular degeneration. I, like every other eye doctor in the world, didn't have answers to questions from patients or their families as to why they developed the disease. We'd say, "It occurs with aging." The only treatment we had to recommend (laser surgery, now rarely used) left behind damaging scar tissue.

Many eye doctors were skeptical when I began my research on nutrition, lifestyle, and macular degeneration. At scientific meetings, my talks were scheduled near lunchtime, and moderators would joke about the study of diet and eye disease. Then, from 1994 to 1996, we reported that the antioxidant nutrients lutein and zeaxanthin, which are also called carotenoids (abundant in spinach and kale), along with the anti-inflammatory nutrients called omega-3 long-chain polyunsaturated fatty acids (found in salmon, sardines, herring, and mackerel), could reduce the risk of macular degeneration, the leading cause of vision loss among the elderly. We discovered that 6,000 µg of lutein and 2,000 µg of zeaxanthin per day from food sources like spinach and summer squash could reduce the risk of macular degeneration by 43 percent and 2 or more servings per week of fish (rich in omega-3 fatty acids) could reduce the risk by 40 percent.

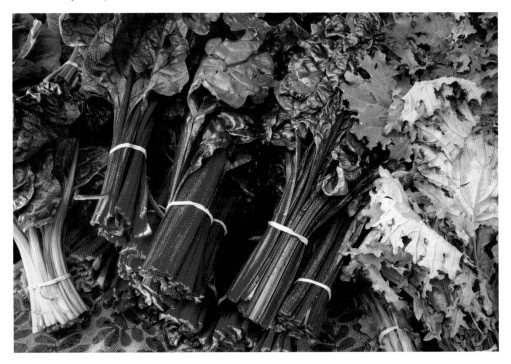

Fortunately, today we know much more about how to prevent and slow the progression of eye diseases such as macular degeneration: don't smoke; exercise regularly; maintain a normal weight; eat a diet that is anti-inflammatory and rich in antioxidants; maintain normal blood pressure, cholesterol, and blood sugar; and protect your eyes (and skin!) from extreme or prolonged exposure to sun. Widely replicated, our findings are incorporated routinely into the medical management of patients: they are informed that foods rich in antioxidants and a healthy lifestyle can reduce the progression of macular degeneration and possibly cataracts, and that foods rich in omega-3 fatty acids can help ward off the advanced forms of this disease and possibly others that damage the retinal layer of the eye and cause loss of vision. Lutein and zeaxanthin pigments are found naturally in the macula (the central part of the retina) and omega-3 fatty acids are found in abundance in rods and cones, the light receptors that enable us to see. So we have learned that we are indeed what we eat.

Of course, knowledge, awareness, and good intentions don't always change habits—anyone who's ever failed at a New Year's resolution knows this. So here is what I propose to everyone who wants to maintain healthy vision: shop, cook, and eat from this book for three meals a day (if possible) for the next four weeks. During that month, you will experience new delicious meals, and in another month eating them routinely may become second nature. Use this cookbook to inspire you to create other recipes with eye-healthy foods. These habits could last you a lifetime.

My macular degeneration patients often lament that they cannot see faces. I want you to see faces, especially the faces of people you love.

Johanna M. Seddon, MD, ScM
Professor, Tufts University School of Medicine
Director, Tufts Medical Center Ophthalmic
Epidemiology and Genetics Service

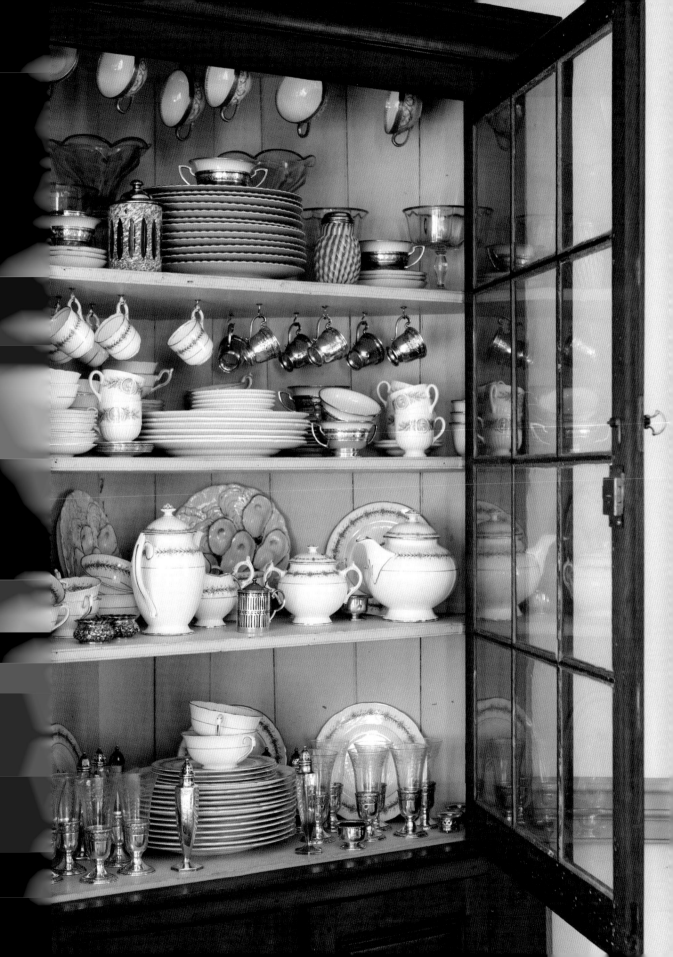

Getting Started

Remember your mother telling you to eat carrots for good eyesight? She was right. Today we've learned that not only carrots, but also a host of other vegetables, fish, nuts, and fruits can affect your eye health. Indeed, not just the foods, but also their pairing combinations—tomatoes with olive oil, avocados with pink grapefruit—can have a positive impact. If you are among the ten million Americans with age-related macular degeneration, which may cause 1 out of 4 baby boomers to lose their central vision eventually, eating the right foods may be not only a good idea but also critical to your health.

So, eat your antioxidants. But where does one find flavorful recipes with ingredients customized to benefit your eyes? We can't live on carrot soup. Health cookbooks on the market tend to be uninspired, with recipes that are often dull and bland. Beautiful lifestyle cookbooks—the

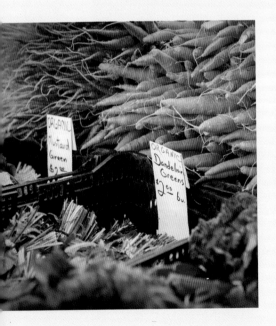

ones we savor and pore over—often have enough salt and fat to give you high blood pressure. What's been missing is a savory cookbook that's fun to read (easy on the eyes) while also highlighting ingredients that promote eye well-being. Assembled here for the first time is a cookbook that guides you along the road to good eye health while offering original recipes that taste great too.

It can be hard work figuring out what foods are best for your health and then finding a way to cook them interestingly week after week. For years, I'd rely on a few staples and just eat sensibly, hoping I got everything

I needed. We all know that oranges are a great source of vitamin C and contain an impressive amount of essential nutrients, vitamins, and minerals; many people drink orange juice daily as a result. But who would think to eat sardines, which not only are a power food in staving off macular degeneration, but also pack a nutritional wallop with high omega-3 fatty acids and protein that helps lower blood pressure, reduces the risk of heart attack, and is an important anti-inflammatory agent (essential for healthy skin, hair, and nails)? Moreover, how do you prepare sardines, other than serving them on crackers with mustard? People are busy, and life gets in the way of researching nutritional goals and how to achieve them through diet. This book spells out what you need for healthy eating and dishes up flavor and variety. (One simple hint: eat yellow, red, and green fruits or vegetables every day.)

Our instinct to eat certain foods to promote eye health is not new; in the sixteenth century, Spanish explorers took chile peppers, which are rich in beta-carotene, vitamins C, E, B6, and folic acid, on sea voyages to promote night vision. Ancient Greek philosophers wrote about the medical benefits of olive oil. In the 1920s, the nutritionist Victor Lindlahr (who, as Dr. Seddon notes, was an early believer in the idea that food determines health) developed the Catabolic Diet. That view gained some adherents at the time, with the earliest recorded support coming from an ad in the *Bridgeport Telegraph* in 1923:

> Ninety per cent of the diseases known to man are caused by cheap foodstuffs. You are what you eat.

With this cookbook, we take his advice to heart. Indeed, our hearts, bodies, and eyes depend on it.

Jennifer Trainer Thompson

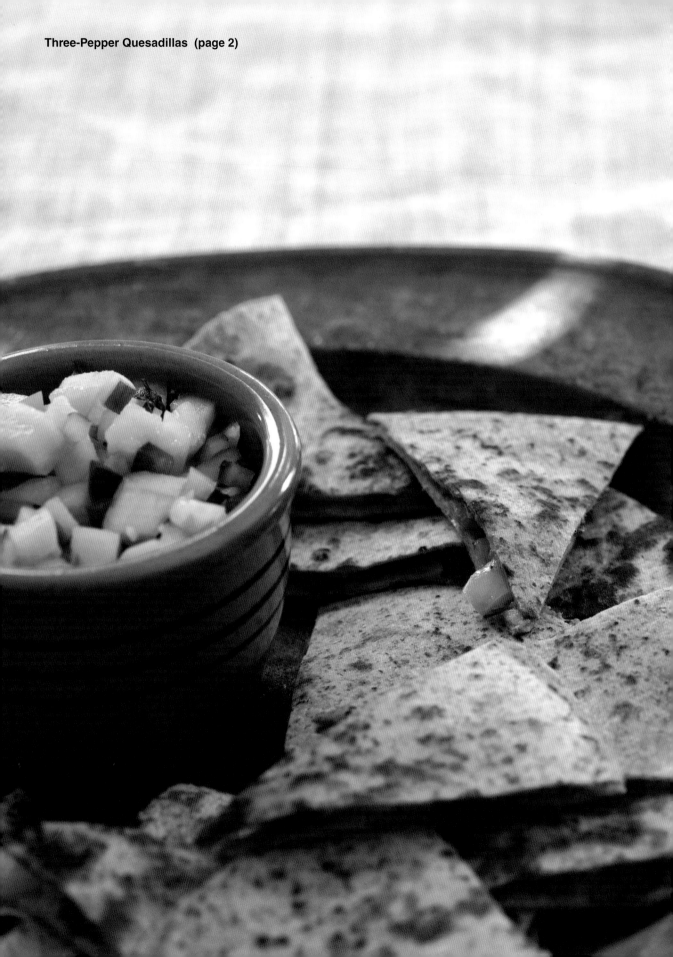

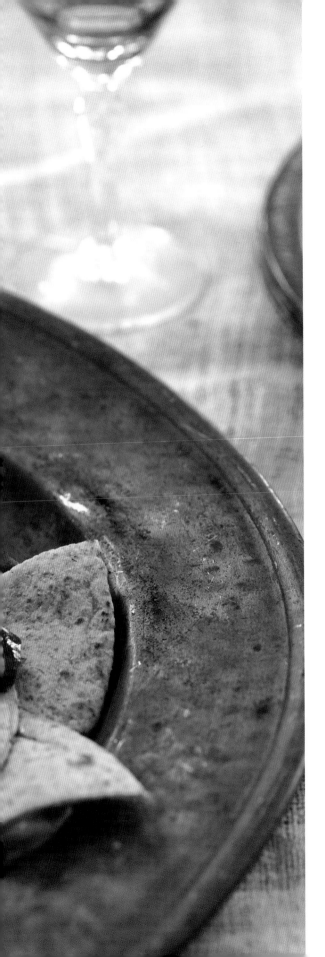

Small Bites

Three-Pepper Quesadillas

Kale Chips

Roasted Butternut
Squash Hummus

Grilled Oysters

Deviled Eggs

Sweet Pea Guacamole

Corn and Sweet Potato Tamales
with Chipotle Sauce

Savory Almonds

Shrimp Cocktail

Smoked Mackerel Dip

Three-Pepper Quesadillas

SERVES 4

Nutritionally dense and high in vitamin C, beta-carotene, and other carotenoids, bell peppers are good for your skin, immune system, and eyes. This recipe is from Roz Torrey, who, with three young children, is skilled at putting together a meal at lightning speed. For variety, add diced zucchini to the peppers, or substitute black beans, corn, and cilantro.

1 tablespoon olive oil

1 cup chopped yellow bell pepper

1 cup chopped red bell pepper

1 cup chopped green or orange bell pepper

½ cup chopped scallions

½ teaspoon ground cumin

½ teaspoon sea salt

¼ teaspoon freshly ground black pepper

¼ teaspoon red pepper flakes or cayenne, or to taste

8 large tortillas (corn or wheat)

1 cup grated cheddar cheese

Heat the oil in a large skillet over medium heat, add the peppers, and sauté until soft, about 10 minutes. Transfer into a bowl and combine with the scallions, cumin, salt, pepper, and red pepper flakes.

> "Did you ever stop to taste a carrot? Not just eat it, but taste it? You can't taste the beauty and energy of the earth in a Twinkie." — *Astrid Alauda*

Heat a second large skillet over medium heat. Add 1 tortilla, and top with ¼ cup bell pepper mixture. Sprinkle with ¼ cup cheese, top with a second tortilla, and cook 2 minutes on each side, or until golden, pressing down with spatula. Repeat with the remaining tortillas, bell pepper mixture, and cheese.

Cut into thin wedges and serve.

Nutritional Profile

Serving size: 1 quesadilla

Calories: 282
Protein: 11 g
Fiber: 5 g
Fat: 14 g
Saturated fat: 7 g
Sodium: 553 mg
Vitamin A: 1,593 IU
Vitamin C: 150 mg
Vitamin D: 7 IU
Vitamin E: 2 IU
Beta-carotene: 726 µg
Lutein and zeaxanthin: 276 µg

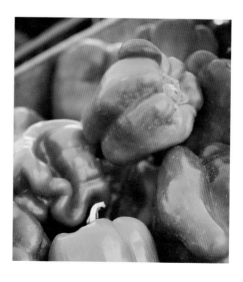

Kale Chips

Raw kale has an exceptional nutrient profile, with the highest content of lutein of any vegetable, as well as zeaxanthin (antioxidants found in the macula). Kale is also rich in vitamin K (the "k" comes from the German *koagulation,* or "coagulation" in English), which helps promote bone health and assists the liver in generating blood-clotting proteins. One cup of chopped kale gives you 1,000 micrograms of vitamin K—10 times the suggested daily dose.

- 8   cups loosely packed kale, stems removed
- 2   tablespoons olive oil
- ½   teaspoon sea salt
- ¼   teaspoon smoked paprika
- ¼   teaspoon garlic powder
- ¼   teaspoon onion powder
- ⅛   teaspoon freshly ground black pepper

Preheat the oven to 325°F. Wash and dry the kale and tear it into large pieces.

Place the dried kale in a bowl and toss to coat with oil. Spread it out on a baking sheet lined with parchment. Bake until crispy but not burnt, 20 to 25 minutes.

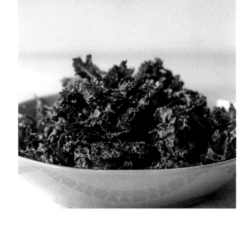

To make the seasoning, combine the remaining ingredients in a small bowl. Sprinkle the seasoning over the kale chips and serve.

Note: If you are taking anticoagulant medication, check with your doctor about intake of green, leafy vegetables and eat them in small to moderate amounts at regular intervals rather than irregularly in large amounts.

Nutritional Profile

Serving size: 1 cup

Calories: 100
Protein: 2 g
Fiber: 5 g
Fat: 8 g
Saturated fat: 1 g
Sodium: 363 mg
Vitamin A: 2,954 IU
Vitamin C: 50 mg
Vitamin E: 2 IU
Beta-carotene: 1,768 µg
Lutein and zeaxanthin: 1,633 µg
Omega-3 fatty acids: 1 g

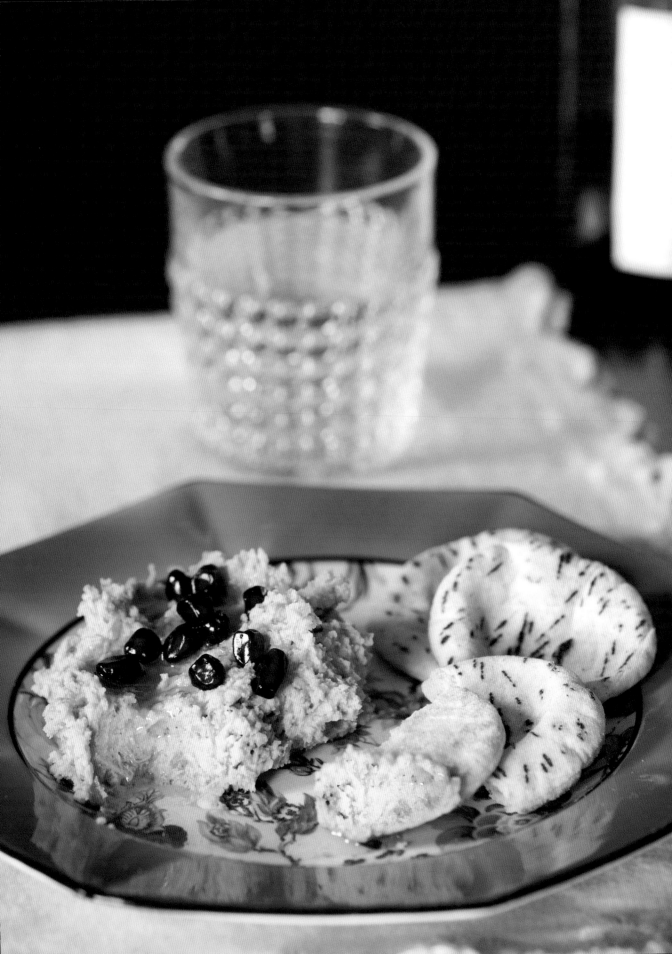

Roasted Butternut Squash Hummus

MAKES 3 CUPS

Squash is rich in carotenoids. You might dress up this dish by drizzling the top of the hummus with a little extra virgin olive oil, chopped cilantro, chopped walnuts, and pomegranate seeds. Serve with warm whole wheat pita triangles or flour tortillas for lunch, brunch, a snack, or an appetizer.

1	small butternut squash, peeled, seeded, and cut into 2-inch chunks (about 2 cups)
1	tablespoon plus 2 tablespoons extra virgin olive oil
One	15-ounce can chickpeas, drained
¼	cup tahini
3	tablespoons freshly squeezed lemon juice
¼	teaspoon ground coriander
½	teaspoon ground cumin
1	tablespoon freshly chopped cilantro
3	garlic cloves, minced
1	teaspoon hot sauce
½	teaspoon sea salt
	Freshly ground black pepper
⅛	teaspoon cayenne, more for serving

CONTINUED

Preheat the oven to 350°F. Toss the squash with 1 tablespoon of olive oil, place on a baking sheet, and roast until the squash is tender, about 30 minutes. Set aside to cool.

In a food processor, pulse the chickpeas until coarsely chopped, then add the cooked squash, tahini, lemon juice, coriander, cumin, cilantro, garlic, hot sauce, salt, and pepper; process until smooth.

To serve, ladle the mixture into a bowl, drizzle with the remaining 2 tablespoons of olive oil, and dust with cayenne.

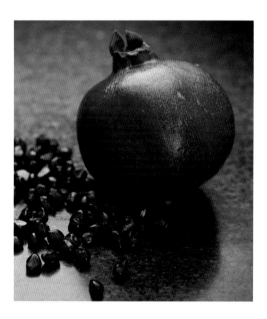

Nutritional Profile

Serving size: 2 tablespoons

Calories: 64

Protein: 2 g

Fiber: less than 1 g

Fat: 4 g

Sodium: 105 mg

Vitamin A: 1,254 IU

Vitamin C: 3 mg

Vitamin E: 1 IU

Beta-carotene: 498 µg

Lutein and zeaxanthin: 2 µg

Grilled Oysters

SERVES 4

A taste for oyster is one worth acquiring. A great source of protein, oysters also have a lot of zinc, which works to assist the conversion of vitamin A into a usable form and helps your body transport the vitamin through your blood. In addition, zinc ensures proper release of the vitamin from the stores held in your liver.

SAUCE

¼   cup (½ stick) unsalted butter

Pinch of kosher salt

Freshly ground black pepper

1   garlic clove, minced

Pinch of cayenne

2   teaspoons freshly squeezed lemon juice

1   teaspoon freshly chopped parsley

24   oysters, on the half shell

⅓   cup bread crumbs

½   cup mixed grated Romano and Parmesan cheeses,

Hot sauce, for serving

CONTINUED

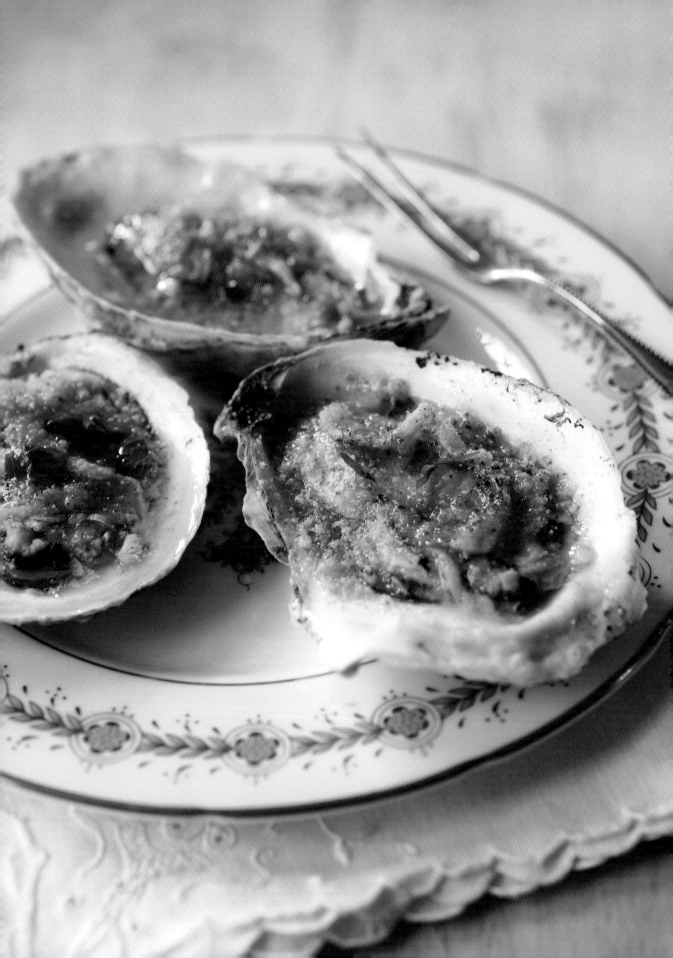

To make the sauce, melt the butter in a saucepan, add the other ingredients, and stir to blend. Keep warm.

Preheat a grill to medium-high heat. Place the oysters on the grill, cover, and cook until the edges start to curl, about 4 minutes.

Top each oyster with a generous amount of bread crumbs and cheese and return them to the grill. When the topping bubbles, ladle a little butter sauce on each. Serve the oysters in the shell with hot sauce on the side.

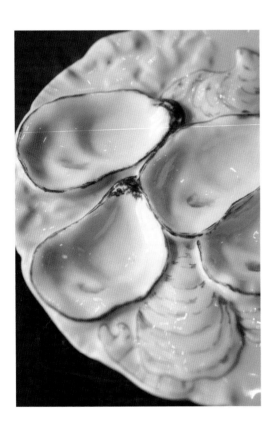

Nutritional Profile

Serving size: 6 oysters

Calories: 457
Protein: 35 g
Fiber: less than 1 g
Fat: 24 g
Saturated fat: 12 g
Sodium: 685 mg
Vitamin A: 1,214 IU
Vitamin D: 8.8 IU
Zinc: 50 mg
Beta-carotene: 52 µg
Lutein and zeaxanthin: 26 µg
Omega-3 fatty acids: 8.5 g

Deviled Eggs

SERVES 6

The devil is in the details, and after getting a bad rap for years, eggs have come roaring back, for good reason: they are loaded with protein, vitamins, and minerals. The yolk of the egg also boasts carotenoids, including lutein and zeaxanthin.

6   hard-boiled eggs (see page 14)

3   tablespoons mayonnaise

1   teaspoon Dijon mustard

1   teaspoon hot sauce or curry powder

1   teaspoon freshly chopped basil

    Sea salt

    Freshly ground black pepper

    Smoked paprika, for garnish

Peel and slice the eggs lengthwise. Remove the yolks without breaking the whites.

With a fork, gently crush the yolks in a mixing bowl with the mayonnaise, mustard, hot sauce and basil, mixing well. Season to taste with salt and pepper.

Using a teaspoon, mound the mixture lightly into the egg whites and dust each egg with paprika.

Nutritional Profile

Serving size: 1 egg

Calories: 109

Protein: 6 g

Fiber: less than 1 g

Fat: 8 g

Saturated fat: 2 g

Sodium: 368 mg

Vitamin A: 383 IU

Vitamin D: 44 IU

Vitamin E: 1 IU

Beta-carotene: 70 µg

Lutein and zeaxanthin: 228 µg

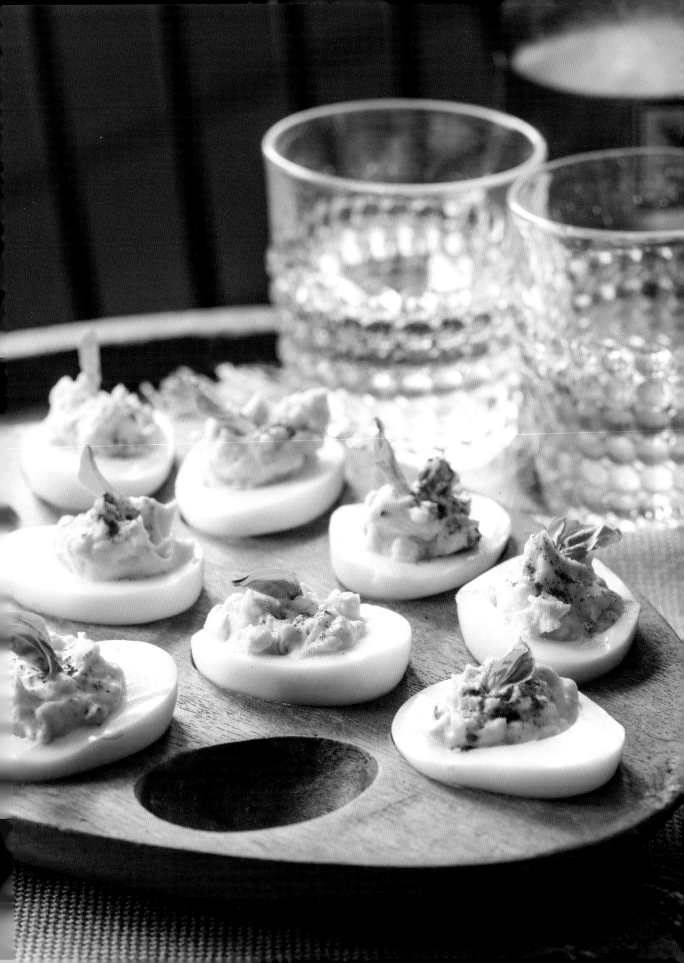

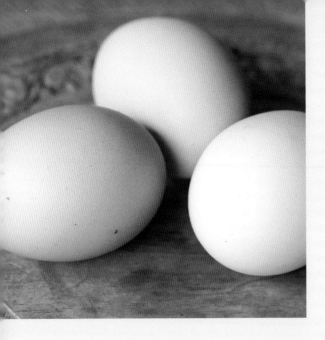

How to Hard-Boil Eggs

To hard-boil eggs, place them in a saucepan and add water to cover them by 1 inch. Bring to a boil over high heat. Remove from the heat, cover and let stand for 12 minutes. Drain the eggs and rinse them under cold running water. Set aside to cool completely. To peel the eggs, once they have cooked and cooled, tap each egg gently on the counter or sink all over to crackle it. Roll the egg between your hands to loosen the shell. Peel, starting at the large end, while holding the egg under running cold water; this facilitates peeling and also removes any stray shell fragments.

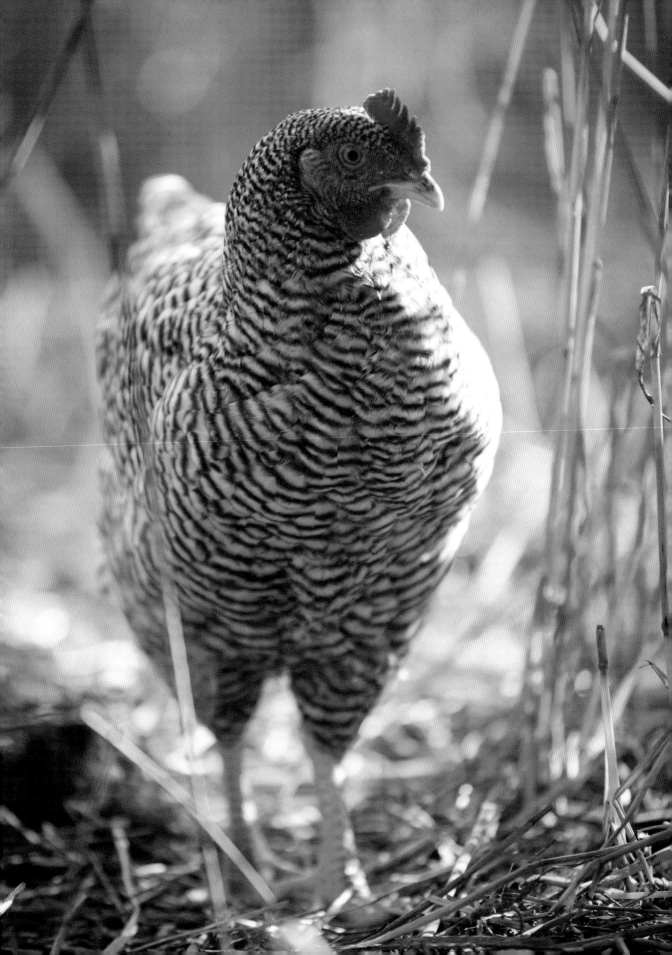

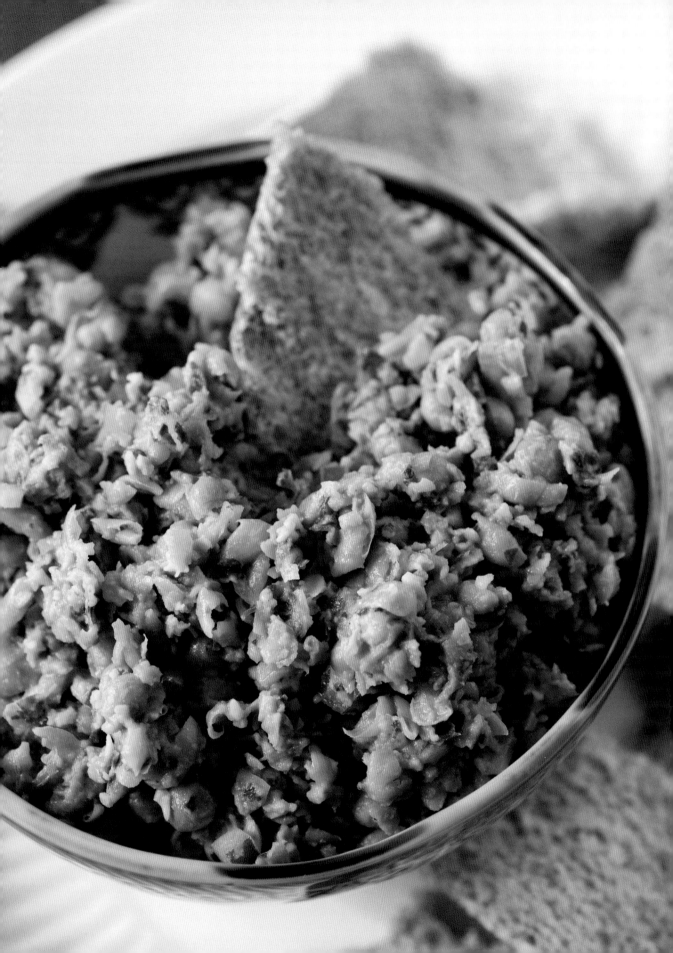

Sweet Pea Guacamole

MAKES 2 CUPS

Peas have antioxidant and anti-inflammatory benefits, and they are environmentally friendly, too. This fresh-tasting guacamole has a subtle pea flavor, enough garlic to get noticed, and a gorgeous bright green color that doesn't fade—perfect to set out before a party. Serve with homemade pita chips or spread on a sandwich.

2	tablespoons extra virgin olive oil
2	tablespoons freshly squeezed lemon juice
½	cup freshly chopped cilantro
¼	cup freshly chopped parsley
1	garlic clove, minced
½	teaspoon hot sauce
12	ounces frozen peas (2 heaping cups), thawed
¼	teaspoon ground cumin
¾	teaspoon sea salt
¼	teaspoon freshly ground black pepper
¼	cup chopped red onion, for garnish

Nutritional Profile

Serving size: 2 tablespoons

Calories: 93
Protein: 3 g
Fiber: 3 g
Fat: 5 g
Saturated fat: 1 g
Sodium: 424 mg
Vitamin A: 1,391 IU
Vitamin C: 17 mg
Vitamin E: 1 IU
Beta-carotene: 829 µg
Lutein and zeaxanthin: 1,478 µg

Combine the olive oil, lemon juice, cilantro, parsley, garlic, and hot sauce in a blender and process until roughly puréed. Add the peas, cumin, salt, and pepper. Blend until puréed but still textured. Pour into a bowl and garnish with the red onion.

Note: For homemade pita chips, using a knife or a pair of scissors, open a pita, then cut it into wedges. Brush the inside of each wedge with olive oil. Sprinkle with salt and pepper (or thyme or rosemary) and broil on a baking sheet to desired crispness.

Corn and Sweet Potato Tamales with Chipotle Sauce

MAKES 10 TAMALES

Sweet potatoes are rich in beta-carotene, which enhances our immune function and may enhance eye health. One cup of sweet potatoes has seven times the daily recommended amount of vitamin A. Masa harina is a type of corn flour used in Mexican cooking and can be found in health food stores or Mexican markets.

12	medium dried corn husks
1	sweet potato
¼	cup (½ stick) unsalted butter
½	cup lightly packed grated cheddar cheese
¾	cup masa harina
¼	teaspoon baking powder
	Pinch of sea salt
1½	cups fresh corn kernels
	Freshly ground black pepper
1	teaspoon chili, ancho, or chipotle powder
1	roasted red bell pepper (see page 21), peeled, seeded, and diced
2	tablespoons chopped scallions
	Chipotle Sauce (see page 22)

CONTINUED

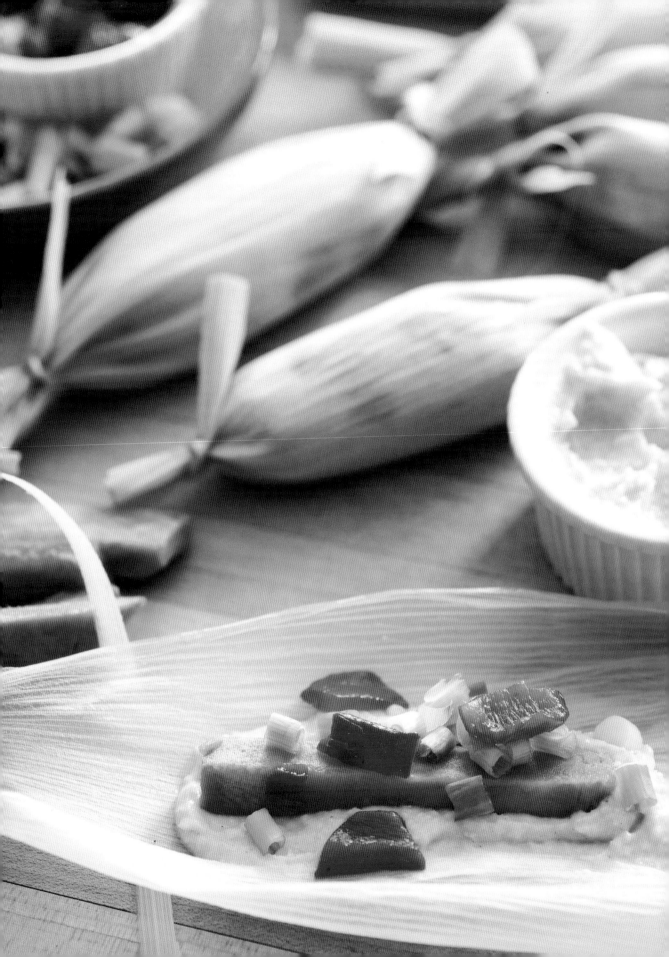

Soak the corn husks in ⅓ cup of warm water until flexible (a few hours).

Preheat the oven to 450°F. Peel the sweet potato if desired and cut in half lengthwise, then cut into ¼-inch half moons. Place on a rimmed baking sheet sprayed with nonstick cooking spray and roast until tender, about 20 minutes, turning after 10 minutes. Remove from oven and set aside.

Drain the husks. Use several of the longer husks to make ties by tearing off fifteen ⅛-inch-wide strips. Cover with a damp cloth.

With a hand mixer, beat the butter in a bowl until it is fluffy. Add the cheese gradually, beating again until fluffy. In a separate bowl, combine the masa harina, baking powder, and salt. Drizzle in the water slowly (you may not need it all), all the while working the mixture, until a stiff dough forms.

Purée the corn, black pepper, and chili powder in a food processor. Add the masa dough by the spoonful (as the processor runs) and blend. Add the butter mixture by the spoonful, processing until the mixture is light and fluffy.

To make the tamales, open each husk and spread 2 tablespoons of the dough evenly over the husk. Add a few sweet potato slices and sprinkle with the roasted red pepper and scallions. Wrap up the husks and tie the ends.

Steam the tamales in a metal basket steamer over simmering water until firm, about an hour. To serve, place 1 to 2 tamales on each plate and serve with the Chipotle Sauce.

Nutritional Profile

Serving size: 1 tamale

Calories: 251

Protein: 8 g

Fiber: 5 g

Fat: 9 g

Saturated fat: 4 g

Sodium: 134 mg

Vitamin A: 2,444 IU

Vitamin C: 22 mg

Vitamin E: 1 IU

Zinc: 1 mg

Beta-carotene: 1,279 µg

Lutein and zeaxanthin: 81 µg

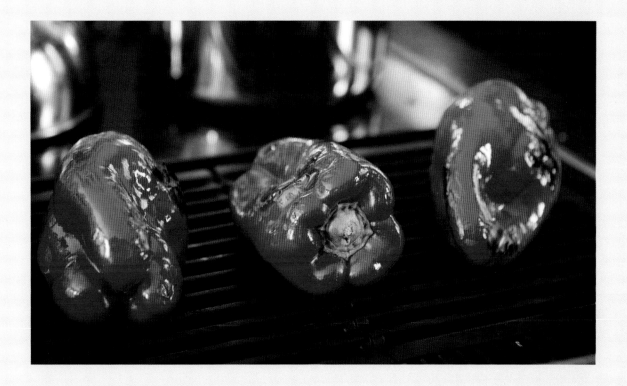

Roasting Red Peppers

You can roast red peppers several ways. If you have just one pepper, hold it with tongs over the flame of a gas stove and char on all sides. If you have several peppers, preheat the oven to 450°F, place the peppers on a rimmed baking sheet and roast, turning every 15 minutes, until done (probably half an hour). Place in a bowl, cover with plastic, and let the steam loosen the skin. Once the peppers have cooled, peel off the blackened skin with a paring knife or your fingers and deseed.

Chipotle Sauce

MAKES 2 CUPS

1	dried chipotle chile
2	teaspoons vegetable oil
1	small yellow onion, finely chopped
2	garlic cloves, minced
½	teaspoon cumin seeds, toasted and ground
¼	teaspoon dried oregano
2	cups tomatoes, peeled, seeded, and chopped (about 2 to 3 large tomatoes)
	Pinch of sea salt
	Freshly ground black pepper

Put the chipotle in a small bowl, cover with hot water, and allow it to soften for 15 minutes. Drain, remove the stem (and seeds if you want a milder sauce), and set aside.

Heat the oil in a saucepan and sauté the onion until soft, about 5 minutes. Add the garlic, cumin, and oregano and cook, stirring occasionally, for 1 minute. Increasing the heat to high, add the tomatoes and chipotle, then reduce heat to low and simmer until slightly thickened, about 20 minutes.

Transfer to a food processor or blender. Purée until smooth. Season to taste. Return to the saucepan and simmer over low heat until heated through, about 5 minutes.

Nutritional Profile

Serving size: ½ cup

Calories: 62
Protein: 1 g
Fiber: 1 g
Fat: 2 g
Sodium: 289 mg
Vitamin A: 242 IU
Vitamin C: 21 mg
Vitamin E: 1 IU
Beta-carotene: 23 µg
Lutein and zeaxanthin: 34 µg

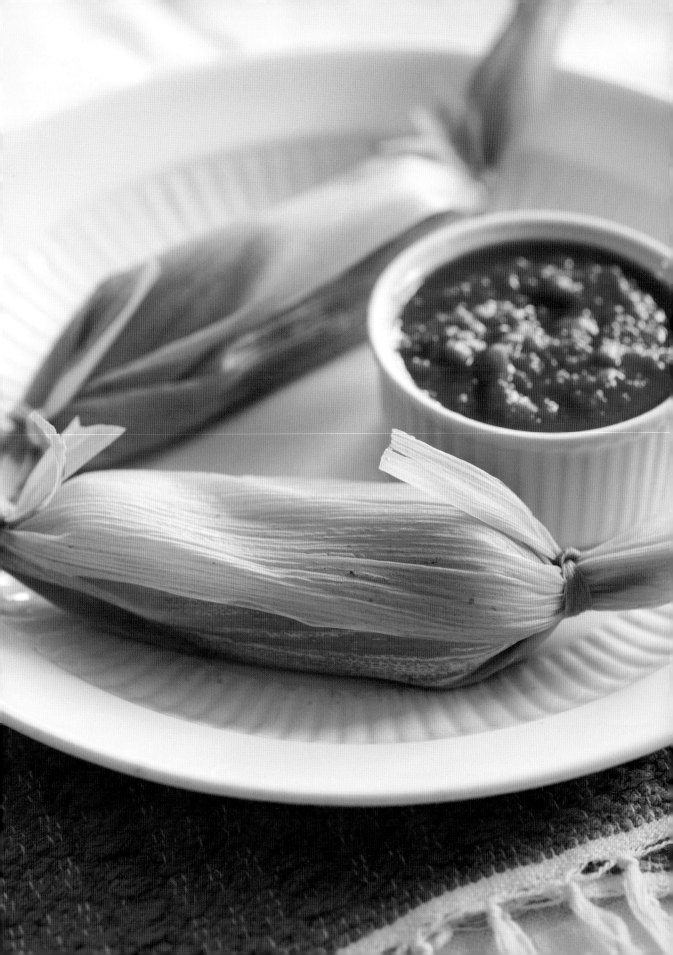

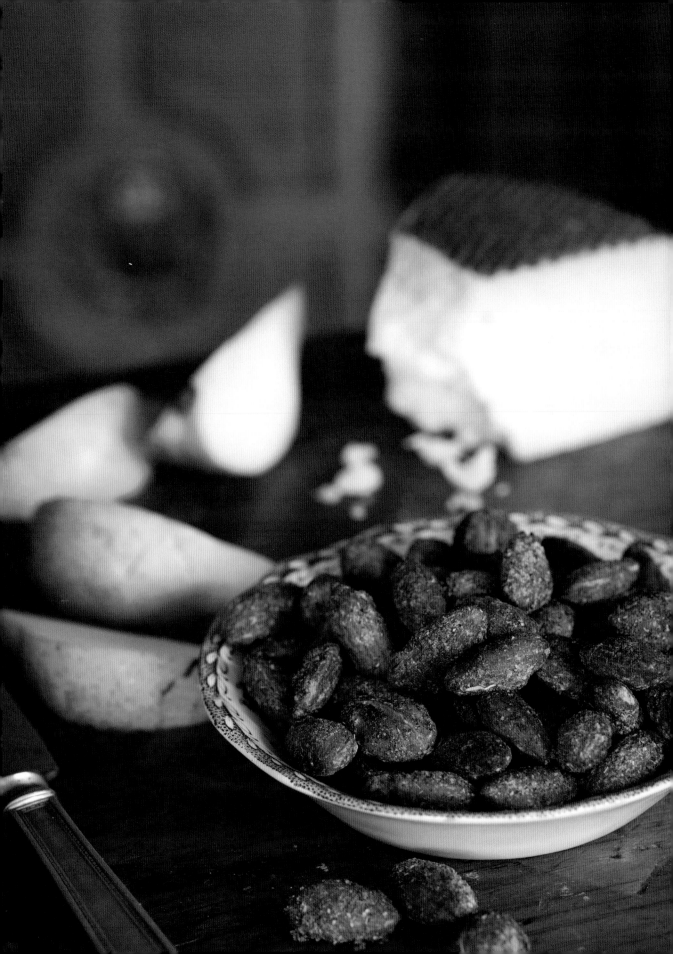

Savory Almonds

Providing fiber, vitamins, and minerals, almonds are a supersnack. These are delicious by themselves, or they can be partnered with slices of ripe pear and shaved Manchego cheese. Almonds are loaded with vitamin E; 22 nuts have 11 IU, or "international units," of vitamin E, which is half the recommended daily allowance.

1	large egg white
4	teaspoons ground cumin
4	teaspoons ground coriander
1	teaspoon ground cardamom
¼	teaspoon ground cloves
½	teaspoon freshly ground black pepper
½	teaspoon sea salt
¼	teaspoon cayenne
2	cups whole unsalted almonds (raw)

Nutritional Profile

Serving size: ½ cup

Calories: 427
Protein: 17 g
Fiber: 10 g
Fat: 35 g
Saturated fat: 3 g
Sodium: 371 mg
Vitamin A: 93 IU
Vitamin E: 28 IU
Zinc: 2 mg
Beta-carotene: 51 µg
Lutein and zeaxanthin: 17 µg

Preheat the oven to 350°F. Using a fork or whisk, beat the egg white in a medium bowl until frothy. Set the bowl aside. Combine the spices in a separate bowl. Toss the almonds in the egg white, then in the spice mix, stirring to blend. Spread the almonds in a single layer on a baking sheet and bake until toasted and lightly browned, 15 to 20 minutes, stirring after 10 minutes. Remove to a rack to cool completely.

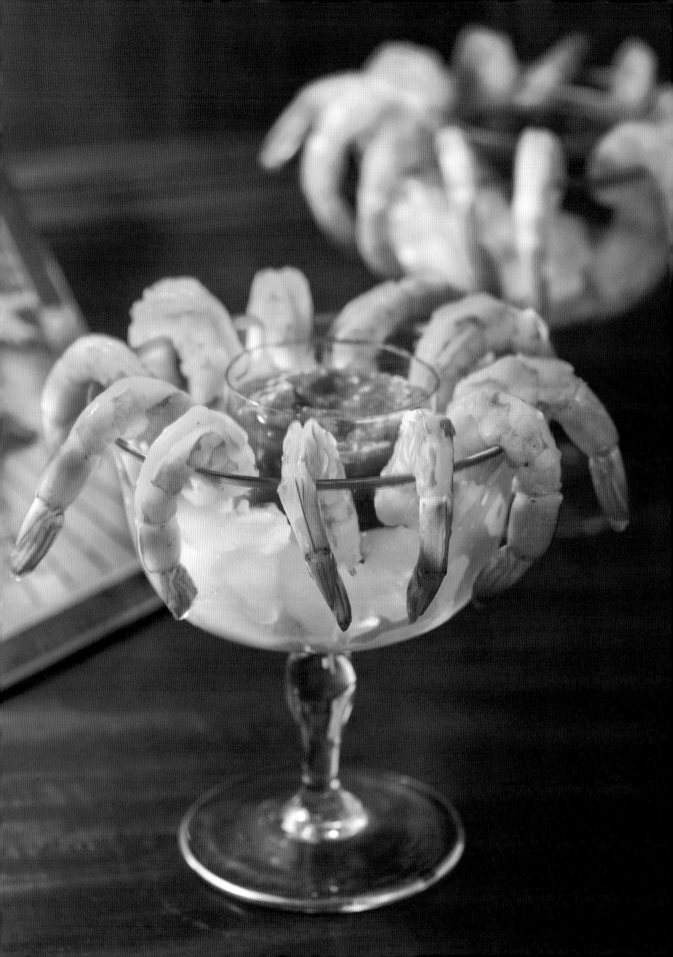

Shrimp Cocktail

SERVES 2 – 4

L ow in calories and saturated fats, but high in essential fats and other nutrients, shrimp are a healthy staple and an excellent source of selenium and protein.

COCKTAIL SAUCE

6	tablespoons ketchup
6	tablespoons Heinz® Chili Sauce
6	tablespoons prepared horseradish
4	teaspoons freshly squeezed lemon juice
1	teaspoon freshly ground black pepper
2	teaspoons hot sauce
1	teaspoon Worcestershire sauce
2	garlic cloves, minced
1	dozen cold cooked large shrimp, deveined, peeled, and with tails
	Lemon wedges, for garnish

Combine the sauce ingredients in a small bowl, taste, season if necessary, then cover and chill for 2 hours before serving. Spoon into martini glasses, then decorate the rims of the glasses with fresh shrimp. Garnish with lemon wedges.

Nutritional Profile

Serving size: 3 shrimp

Calories: 113
Protein: 11 g
Fiber: 2 g
Fat: 4 g
Saturated fat: less than 1 g
Sodium: 931 mg
Vitamin A: 535 IU
Vitamin C: 8.5 mg
Vitamin D: 15 IU
Vitamin E: 1 IU
Beta-carotene: 131 µg
Lutein and zeaxanthin: 7 µg
Lycopene: 3,760 µg

Smoked Mackerel Dip

MAKES 2 CUPS

Like sardines and herring, mackerel is loaded with omega-3 fatty acids, which may reduce your risk of heart disease and help your eyes as well. The Japanese, who have arguably the lowest heart disease rate in the world, eat an average of 21 ounces of fish weekly, whereas Americans eat an average of 7 ounces. In this recipe, you could substitute smoked salmon or bluefish. Serve with vegetables or low-sodium wheat crackers for a healthy, tasty hors d'oeuvre or snack.

8 ounces cream cheese, softened

½ cup sour cream

2 teaspoons freshly squeezed lemon juice

1 teaspoon capers

2 tablespoons finely chopped red onion

4 ounces smoked mackerel, coarsely chopped

Combine the ingredients in a food processor and pulse until blended.

Nutritional Profile

Serving size: ½ cup

Calories: 343

Protein: 10 g

Fiber: less than 1 g

Fat: 32 g

Saturated fat: 17 g

Sodium: 1,480 mg

Vitamin A: 1,009 IU

Vitamin C: 1 mg

Vitamin D: 14 IU

Vitamin E: 1 IU

Zinc: 1 mg

Beta-carotene: 52 µg

Lutein and zeaxanthin: 1 µg

Omega-3 fatty acids: 2 g

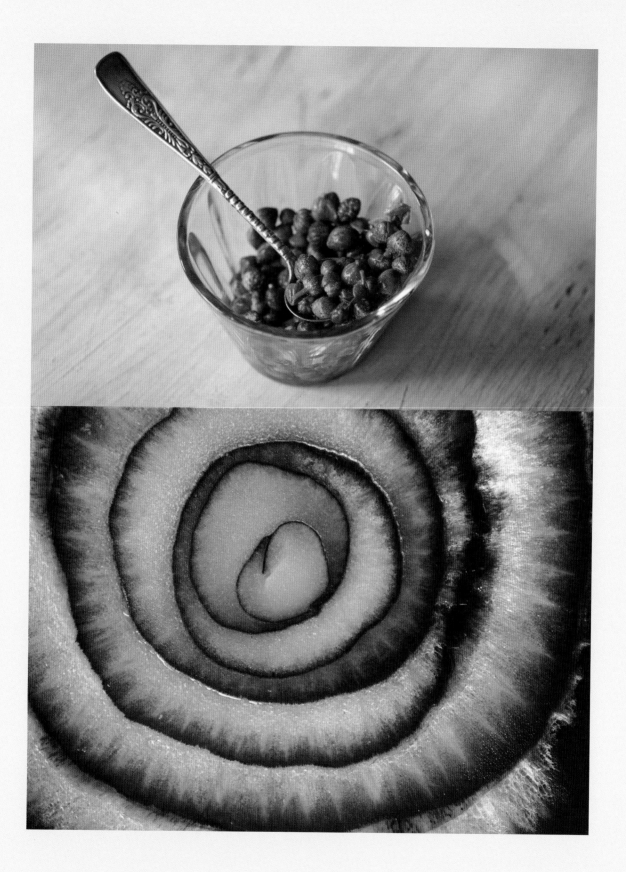

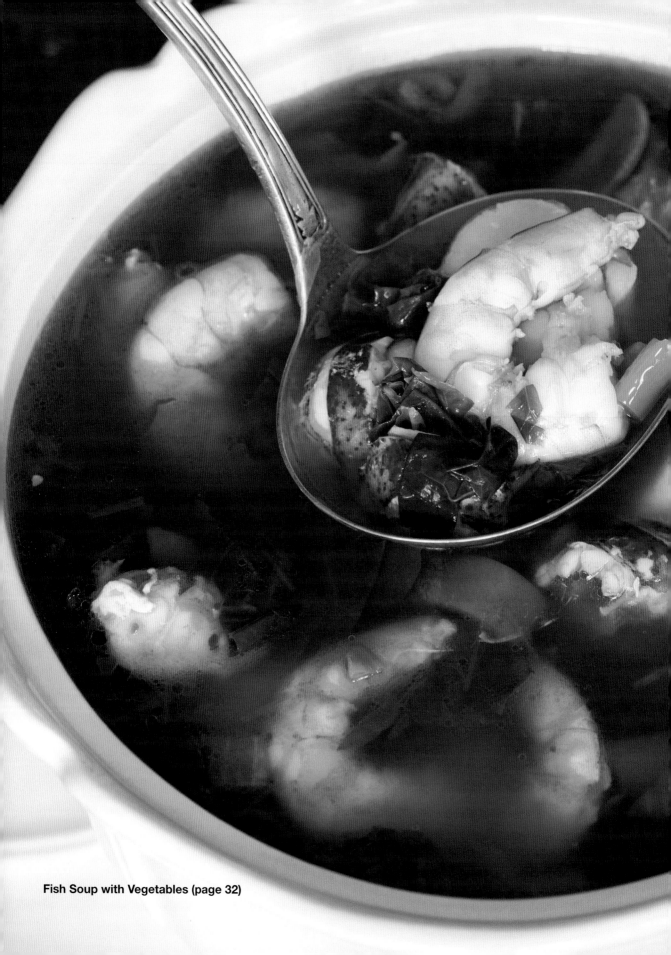

Fish Soup with Vegetables (page 32)

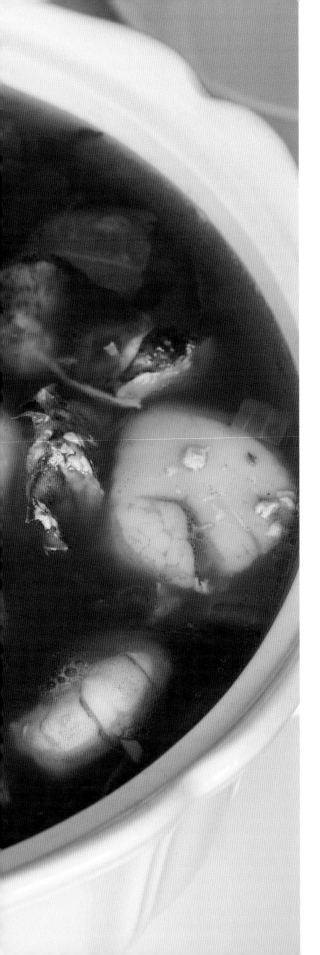

Soups

Fish Soup with Vegetables

T his hearty soup, high in protein from the fish, also packs a wallop from the beta-carotene found in the vegetables. It is from Lidia Matticchio Bastianich, the formidable chef and author of *Lidia Cooks from the Heart of Italy.*

12	ounces monkfish fillet (silver skin removed)
8	ounces sea scallops, preferably "dry" (not soaked in preservatives)
1	pound large shrimp
¼	cup extra virgin olive oil
2	medium onions, chopped (about 2 cups)
5	plump garlic cloves, crushed and peeled
¼	teaspoon peperoncino flakes, or to taste
½	teaspoon plus 1 tablespoon kosher salt
4	Anaheim peppers, seeded and diced (about 2 cups)
1	cup canned Italian plum tomatoes, preferably San Marzano, crushed by hand
6	quarts (24 cups) cold water
1	pound Swiss chard, sliced in ½-inch shreds

Slice the monkfish into ½-inch chunks. Pull off the side muscle or "foot" from the scallops and discard. Remove the shells, tails, and digestive veins from the shrimp; rinse them and pat dry.

> *"Don't eat anything your great-grandmother wouldn't recognize as food."* — *Michael Pollan*

Pour the olive oil into a heavy-bottomed saucepan or soup pot and set it over medium heat. Scatter in the onions, garlic, and peperoncino and season with ½ teaspoon of salt. Cook, stirring occasionally, until the onions are softened and slightly caramelized, about 8 to 10 minutes, then stir in the diced peppers and cook another 3 minutes or so, until the peppers are tender.

Pour in the crushed tomatoes, raise the heat a bit, and cook, stirring, until the tomatoes have dried out, about 3 to 4 minutes. Pour in the water and the remaining tablespoon salt, stir well, cover, and bring the water to a boil over high heat. Adjust the heat to maintain a gentle boil and cook, covered, for an hour; then stir in the Swiss chard shreds. Return the broth to a steady simmer and cook uncovered for 45 minutes, or until the chard is very tender and the broth has reduced to 4 quarts (16 cups).

To finish the soup: add the chunks of monkfish to the simmering broth, cover, and cook for 5 minutes. Drop in the scallops, stir, and simmer for 7 more minutes. Add the shrimp, return the broth to a bubbling simmer, and cook for a minute or two, just until the shrimp are cooked through. Serve immediately in warm shallow soup bowls.

Nutritional Profile

Serving size: 2 cups

Calories: 333
Protein: 47 g
Fiber: 3 g
Fat: 10 g
Saturated fat: 2 g
Sodium: 1,242 mg
Vitamin A: 8,538 IU
Vitamin C: 25 mg
Vitamin D: 202 IU
Vitamin E: 4 IU
Zinc: 2 mg
Beta-carotene: 4,999 µg
Lutein and zeaxanthin: 5,545 µg
Omega-3 fatty acids: 1 g

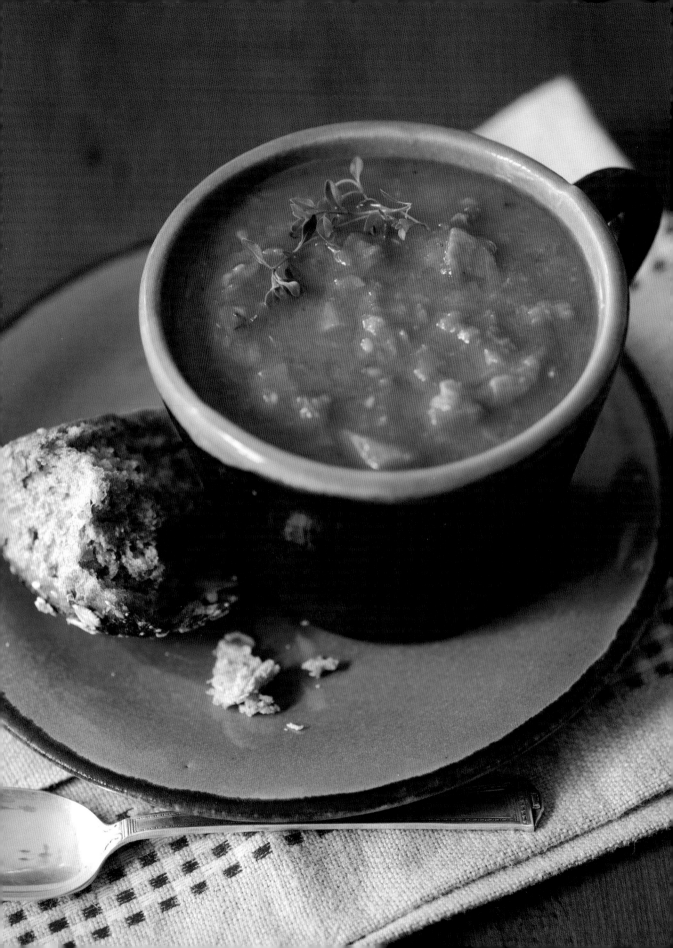

Roasted Tomato and Carrot Soup

SERVES 4–6

Some evidence suggests that cooking may enhance the absorption of the lycopene in tomatoes, so this soup is both warming and extra nutritious.

2	pounds plum tomatoes, cored and cut in half
1	pound medium carrots, peeled and cut into ½-inch pieces
4	garlic cloves, peeled and left whole
1	medium onion, peeled and coarsely chopped
1	tablespoon freshly chopped thyme
¼	cup olive oil
½	teaspoon sea salt
¼	teaspoon freshly ground black pepper
2 to 3	cups homemade chicken stock or reduced-fat, low-sodium chicken broth

Preheat the oven to 450°F. Place the tomatoes, carrots, garlic, onion, and thyme on a rimmed baking sheet pan. Add the olive oil, salt, and pepper, and toss to coat. Bake for 20 to 30 minutes, until the vegetables are tender. Scrape the tomato mixture into a food processor and process until not quite smooth.

Place the puréed mixture in a medium saucepan, add chicken broth, and simmer on medium-low heat for 10 minutes. Season to taste. Serve immediately.

Nutritional Profile

Serving size: 1 cup

Calories: 181
Protein: 3 g
Fiber: 5 g
Fat: 11 g
Saturated fat: 2 g
Sodium: 578 mg
Vitamin A: 16,691 IU
Vitamin C: 33 mg
Vitamin E: 5 IU
Beta-carotene: 8,345 µg
Lutein and zeaxanthin: 457 µg
Lycopene: 4,669 µg

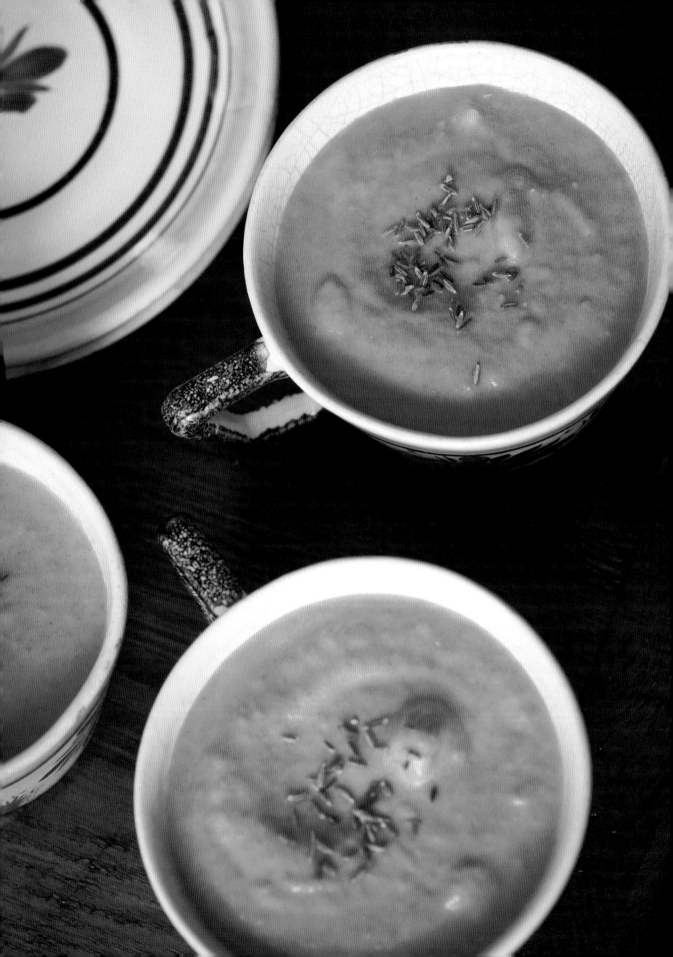

Carrot-Cumin Soup

SERVES 4

A root vegetable with origins in Asia, the carrot is rich in beta-carotene, vitamin A, minerals, and antioxidants. Carrots are one of the highest vegetable sources of vitamin A—two carrots yield roughly four times the recommended daily allowance.

2	tablespoons olive oil
1	medium yellow onion, chopped
2	garlic cloves, minced
1	pound large carrots, peeled and cut into 1-inch pieces (about 2½ cups)
2½	cups vegetable broth
½	teaspoon ground cumin
¼	teaspoon ground coriander
½	teaspoon sea salt
	Freshly ground black pepper
1	teaspoon freshly squeezed lemon juice
½	cup plain Greek yogurt
2	tablespoons toasted cumin seeds, for garnish

Nutritional Profile

Serving size: 1 cup

Calories: 178
Protein: 4 g
Fiber: 4 g
Fat: 11 g
Saturated fat: 3 g
Sodium: 1,031 mg
Vitamin A: 19,312 IU
Vitamin C: 10 mg
Vitamin E: 3 IU
Beta-carotene: 9,420 µg
Lutein and zeaxanthin: 307 µg
Lycopene: 1 µg

In a heavy saucepan, heat the olive oil over medium-high heat and sauté the onion for 2 minutes, then add the garlic and sauté an additional minute. Add the carrots, broth, cumin, coriander, salt, and pepper. Bring to a boil. Reduce the heat, cover, and simmer until the carrots are tender, about 15 minutes.

Purée the soup with an immersion blender or, working in batches, purée in a blender or food processor until smooth, then return it to the saucepan. Whisk in the lemon juice and yogurt. Season to taste. Ladle into bowls and sprinkle with the cumin seeds.

White Bean Soup with Kale

SERVES 4 – 6

Kale turns an ordinary white bean soup into a lutein and zeaxanthin powerhouse. (As a rule, the darker the green, the higher the lutein.) As an alternative, add 6 to 8 ounces of chopped smoked sausage, such as Andouille or chorizo, for a meatier dish with a kick.

2	tablespoons vegetable oil
1½	cups chopped onion
1½	cups chopped carrot
½	cup chopped celery
2	garlic cloves, finely chopped
2	teaspoons freshly chopped thyme
8	cups reduced-sodium chicken or vegetable broth
1½	cups dry navy or great northern beans, soaked overnight
1	teaspoon sea salt
1	teaspoon freshly ground black pepper
4	cups chopped kale leaves, tough stems removed

Heat the oil in a stockpot over medium-high heat. Sauté the onion, carrot, and celery for 7 to 10 minutes, or until softened. Add the garlic and sauté until fragrant, 1 minute. Add the thyme and sauté for 30 seconds. Add the broth, beans, salt, and pepper and stir to combine. Bring to a boil. Reduce the heat, cover, and simmer for 1½ hours, or until the beans are tender, stirring occasionally. Cool slightly.

CONTINUED

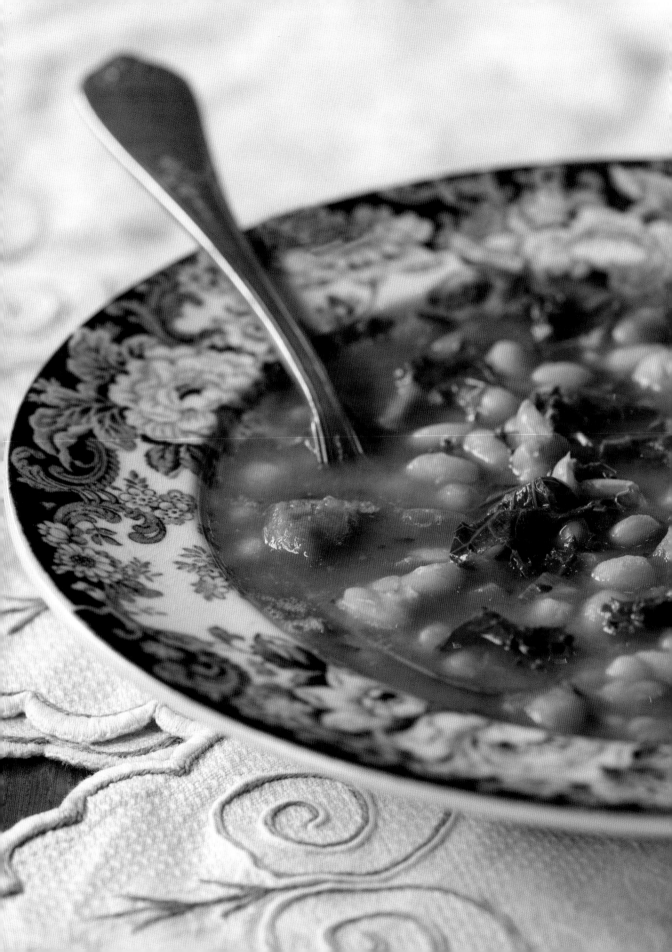

Partially purée the soup with an immersion blender or transfer half the soup to a blender or food processor and purée before adding back to the stockpot. Add the kale and cook for 5 minutes. Season to taste. Ladle into warm bowls and serve immediately.

Nutritional Profile

Serving size: 1 cup

Calories: 357

Protein: 17 g

Fiber: 19 g

Fat: 7 g

Saturated fat: 1 g

Sodium: 847 mg

Vitamin A: 14,721 IU

Vitamin C: 71 mg

Vitamin E: 2 IU

Zinc: 3 mg

Beta-carotene: 8,165 µg

Lutein and zeaxanthin: 21,329 µg

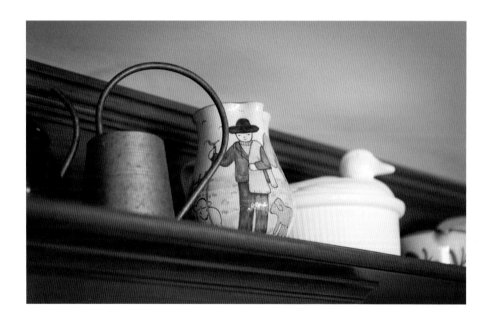

Broccoli Almondine Soup

SERVES 4–6

Almond butter is like peanut butter, but made with almonds, which are more nutritious than peanuts. Choose an all-natural brand made only of ground toasted almonds for the ultimate health benefit. Both broccoli and almonds are high in calcium.

1   teaspoon sea salt

1   pound broccoli florets

2   tablespoons almond butter

¼   cup sun-dried tomatoes packed in olive oil, julienned

Sliced blanched almonds, for garnish

Freshly ground black pepper

Bring 4 cups of water and the salt to a rolling boil in a medium-sized pot on high heat, then add the broccoli. Cover the pot to return it quickly to a boil, cooking the broccoli until stems are easily pierced with a knife, 3 to 4 minutes. Remove from the heat and do not discard the cooking liquid.

Use a slotted spoon to transfer the broccoli to a blender. Add the almond butter and 2 cups of the cooking water. Cover the blender with the lid; remove the steam insert. Cover the hole with a folded paper towel and pulse a few times, allowing steam to escape, then purée until smooth.

Divide the sun-dried tomato among cups or mugs, then pour the soup on top. Garnish with a few almond slices. Season to taste with pepper. Serve immediately.

Nutritional Profile

Serving size: 1 cup

Calories: 119

Protein: 5 g

Fiber: 4 g

Fat: 9 g

Saturated fat: 1 g

Sodium: 606 mg

Vitamin A: 2,746 IU

Vitamin C: 86 mg

Vitamin E: 4 IU

Zinc: 1 mg

Beta-carotene: 15 µg

Lutein and zeaxanthin: 39 µg

Lycopene: 1,240 µg

Roasted Red Pepper Gazpacho

SERVES 4

A Spanish study to analyze the amount of vitamins C and E and carotenoids in commonly eaten foods revealed that only two vegetables contain two thirds of the important nutrients: bell peppers and tomatoes. For maximum effect, work with vegetables that are fully ripe and raw.

2 red bell peppers, roasted (see page 21), peeled and seeded

2 medium tomatoes, cored and diced

1 English cucumber, peeled and diced

1 jalapeño, seeded and minced

6 large radishes, medium-diced

1 garlic clove, minced

½ cup diced red onion

2 cups tomato juice

2 tablespoons freshly chopped cilantro

1 tablespoon freshly squeezed lime juice

¼ teaspoon sea salt

¼ teaspoon ground cumin

Place half the vegetables, along with all the tomato juice, in a blender and purée until smooth. Transfer to a bowl. Add the remaining vegetables, cilantro, lime juice, salt, and cumin and stir to blend. Chill. Season to taste. Serve cold.

Nutritional Profile

Serving size: 1 cup

Calories: 77

Protein: 3 g

Fiber: 3 g

Fat: 1 g

Saturated fat: less than 1 g

Sodium: 527 mg

Vitamin A: 1,554 IU

Vitamin C: 106 mg

Vitamin E: 1 IU

Beta-carotene: 676 µg

Lutein and zeaxanthin: 69 µg

Lycopene: 118 µg

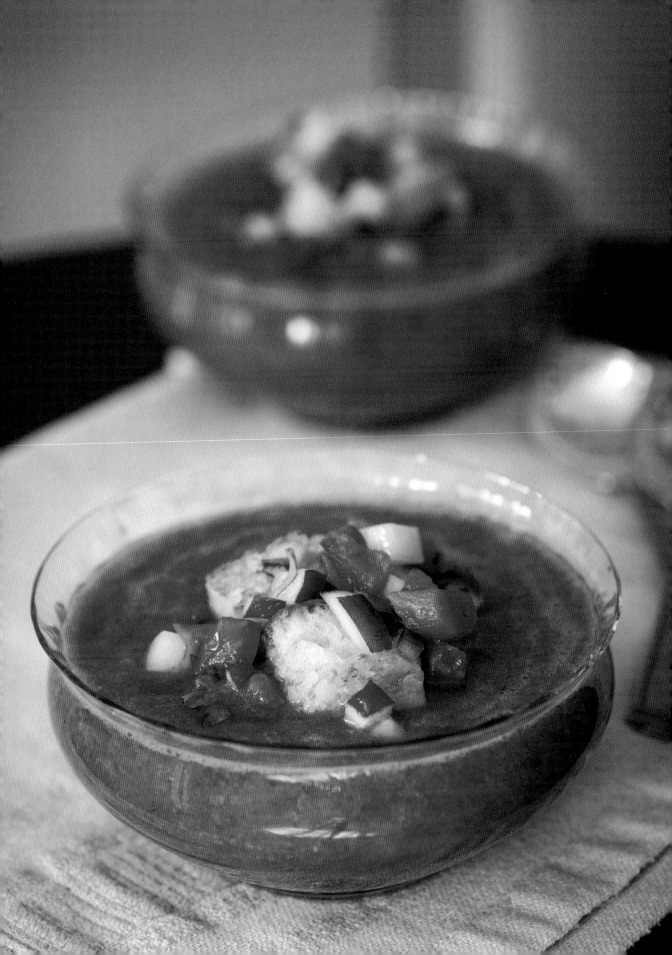

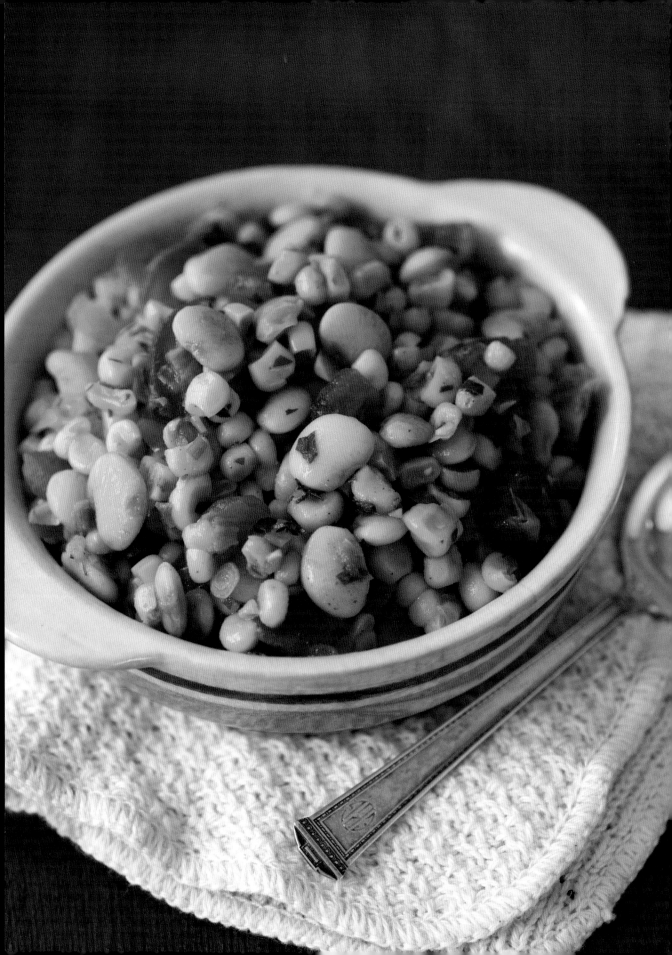

Succotash Ragout

SERVES 4

Innovative, authoritative, and down to earth, Deborah Madison is to vegetarian cooking what Julia Child is to French cooking. This ragout, adapted from her recipe, is made with corn and lima beans, which are high in fiber, folate, and minerals. Serve as a side dish, or with basmati rice for a hearty vegetarian meal.

2 tablespoons olive oil

1 bunch of scallions, including 2 inches of green, sliced thinly

4 cups corn kernels, fresh or frozen

2 cups fresh or one 10-ounce package frozen lima beans

2 tablespoons freshly chopped parsley

2 tablespoons freshly chopped cilantro

1 tablespoon freshly chopped basil

1 teaspoon sea salt

Freshly ground black pepper

½ teaspoon paprika

½ cup vegetable stock

½ cup V8™ juice

2 small tomatoes, seeded and diced

Heat the oil in a wide skillet or sauté pan over medium-high heat. Sauté the scallions, corn, and lima beans for 4 minutes, then add half of the herbs plus the salt, pepper, paprika, stock, and V8™ juice. Simmer for 6 minutes, then add the tomatoes and cook for 2 minutes more, or until they break down. Add the remaining herbs. Season to taste. Serve immediately.

Nutritional Profile

Serving size: 1 cup

Calories: 303

Protein: 10 g

Fiber: 9 g

Fat: 8 g

Saturated fat: 1 g

Sodium: 799 mg

Vitamin A: 1,614 IU

Vitamin C: 36 mg

Vitamin E: 2 IU

Beta-carotene: 818 µg

Lutein and zeaxanthin: 767 µg

Lycopene: 1,171 µg

Green Pea Soup with a Tangerine Twist

SERVES 6

Segments of fresh tangerine (rich in vitamins A and C) lend nutritional heft to this unusual spring soup. Choosing low-sodium or homemade vegetable broth allows you to add salt to your preference.

2½	tablespoons unsalted butter, divided
2	medium leeks, white and light green parts only, thinly sliced and well washed
¼	teaspoon sea salt, plus more to taste
1	quart (4 cups) low-sodium vegetable broth
4	cups fresh or frozen green peas (about 1 pound), divided
½	cup lightly packed fresh mint leaves, chopped
2	tangerines (see Preparing Citrus Fruit, page 49)
4	scallions, thinly sliced
¼	cup low-fat or fat-free plain Greek yogurt
1	tablespoon freshly chopped chives, for garnish

CONTINUED

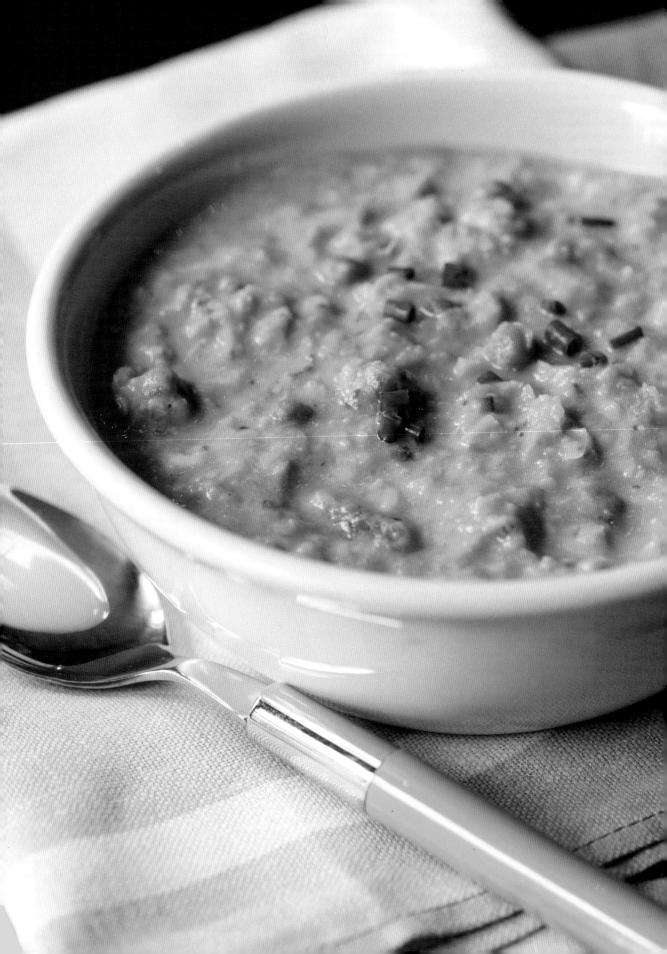

Heat 2 tablespoons of the butter in a saucepan over medium heat. Add the leeks, sprinkle with salt, cover, and cook until tender, about 7 minutes. Uncover and add the vegetable broth, turn up the heat to high, and bring to a boil. Add 3½ cups of the peas. Return to a boil and cook until just tender (about 3 minutes for frozen, 5 minutes for fresh).

Remove from the heat and add the mint leaves. Working in 2 batches, transfer the mixture to a blender. Remove the insert from the lid of the blender and cover the hole with a folded paper towel. Pulse once or twice and then purée. Season to taste. Let rest until ready to serve.

To serve, return the saucepan to medium heat. Add the remaining ½ tablespoon of butter. When the butter is melted, add the scallions and reserved ½ cup of peas and cook 1 minute.

Add the fruit segments, taking care not to break them, and the juice. Swirl to combine and then add the puréed pea mixture. Gently warm; do not bring to a simmer. Gently stir in the yogurt. Season to taste. Spoon into bowls and sprinkle each serving with chopped chives.

Nutritional Profile
Serving size: 1 cup
Calories: 173
Protein: 7 g
Fiber: 7 g
Fat: 5 g
Saturated fat: 3 g
Sodium: 304 mg
Vitamin A: 3,441 IU
Vitamin C: 32 mg
Vitamin D: 4 IU
Vitamin E: 1 IU
Zinc: 1 mg
Beta-carotene: 1,519 µg
Lutein and zeaxanthin: 2,821 µg

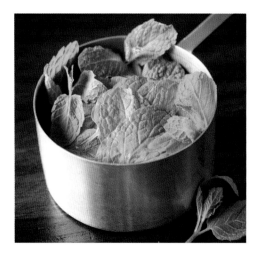

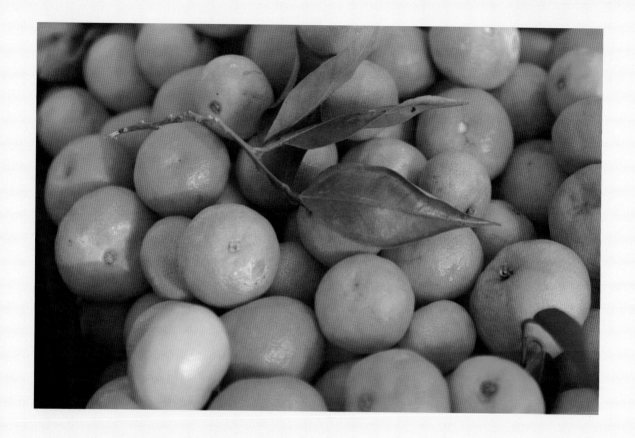

Preparing Citrus Fruit

Using a sharp knife, slice off the top and bottom of each fruit. Following the curve of the fruit, cut away the peel and pith. Hold the fruit over a bowl and cut along both sides of each segment, dividing each segment into quarters, staying as close as possible to the membrane, to release it into the bowl. Before discarding the membrane, squeeze any remaining juice into the bowl with the segments. Remove any seeds. Repeat with the remaining fruit.

Thai Winter Squash Stew

SERVES 4

Many people roll their eyes when tofu is mentioned, but it's high in protein and low in saturated fat, so we're often on the lookout for new (good!) ways to use it. Serve this stew over basmati or jasmine rice. To reduce salt content, garnish with unsalted peanuts.

2	tablespoons olive oil
2	medium leeks, white parts only, thinly sliced and well washed (about 2 cups)
1	tablespoon peeled and minced fresh ginger
3	garlic cloves, minced
2	serrano chiles, stemmed, seeded, and minced
1	tablespoon curry powder
1	tablespoon brown sugar
3	tablespoons light soy sauce
1½	pounds butternut squash, peeled and cut into ½-inch cubes (4 cups)
One	13.5-ounce can coconut milk
½	teaspoon sea salt
¼	teaspoon freshly ground black pepper
One	14-ounce package extra firm tofu, drained and cut into small cubes
	Juice of 1 lime
⅓	cup chopped unsalted peanuts, for garnish
⅓	cup chopped fresh cilantro, for garnish

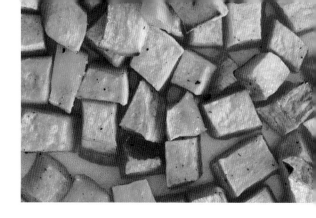

Heat 1 tablespoon of the oil in a sauté pan over medium-high heat. Add the leeks and sauté for 3 minutes. Add the ginger, garlic, and serranos. Sauté until fragrant, about 1 minute. Stir in the curry powder, brown sugar, and soy sauce. Add the squash, coconut milk, salt, pepper, and 1 cup of water and bring to a boil, then reduce to a simmer. Simmer until the squash is tender, about 15 minutes.

Meanwhile, in a large nonstick frying pan, heat the remaining tablespoon of oil over medium-high heat, add the tofu, and sauté until golden brown, about 12 minutes, stirring occasionally.

Add the sautéed tofu and the lime juice to the squash mixture and simmer for a minute. Serve over rice, garnishing with the chopped peanuts and cilantro.

Nutritional Profile

Serving size: 1 cup

Calories: 521

Protein: 15 g

Fiber: 7 g

Fat: 38 g

Saturated fat: 22 g

Sodium: 1,245 mg

Vitamin A: 19,249 IU

Vitamin C: 49 mg

Vitamin E: 7 IU

Zinc: 2 mg

Beta-carotene: 7,888 µg

Lutein and zeaxanthin: 1,286 µg

Miso Soup

SERVES 4

Miso is a fermented soybean paste that has been a staple in the Chinese and Japanese diet for over 2,000 years. Many people in Japan begin their day with a bowl of miso soup, thought to aid digestion and help detoxify the body. Miso is dissolved slowly into a hot soup base called dashi—a light, smoky fish stock made from kelp and dried bonito flakes. Although dashi is easy to make, most people opt for a dried powder that comes in premeasured packets called *hondashi*. This recipe is by Debra Samuels, author of *My Japanese Table*.

- 2 tablespoons dried wakame seaweed
- 4 cups dashi stock (recipe follows, or use packets of dashi powder and follow directions; vegetarian stock is also very good)
- ¼ cup white (mellow) miso
- Half 8-ounce block (250 grams) soft (silken) tofu, cut into 1-inch cubes
- 1 scallion, chopped finely

Add the wakame and 1 cup of water to a large bowl. Set aside for 10 minutes, or until the seaweed is softened. Drain the seaweed, rinse with cold water, and chop coarsely. Set aside.

Bring the dashi to a simmer in a medium saucepan over medium heat, about 3 minutes.

Nutritional Profile

Serving size: 1 cup

Calories: 164

Protein: 15 g

Fiber: 7 g

Fat: 5 g

Saturated fat: 1 g

Sodium: 1,760 mg

Vitamin A: 872 IU

Vitamin C: 4 mg

Vitamin E: 1 IU

Zinc: 1 mg

Beta-carotene: 32 µg

Lutein and zeaxanthin: 43 µg

Place the miso in a ladle. Submerge the ladle about one third of the way into the hot dashi. With a pair of chopsticks or a spoon, dilute the miso, little by little, into the dashi until dissolved.

Add the tofu and seaweed and heat for about 2 minutes. Remove from the heat. Add the scallion and serve immediately.

Dashi Stock

MAKES 4½ CUPS

Dashi stock is the cornerstone of Japanese soups, sauces and many dishes. You can find these ingredients at a well-stocked supermarket or at an Asian grocery.

Two   5-inch strips kombu (dashi kelp)

2½   cups (20 grams) katsuo flakes

Add 4 cups water and the kombu to a medium-size pan. Let the kombu sit in the water for 20 minutes. Then bring the water and kombu to a boil over medium heat. Remove the kombu.

Toss the katsuo flakes into the boiling water and turn off the heat. Let the flakes sit for 2 to 3 minutes, or until they sink to the bottom of the pot.

Set a tightly woven mesh strainer over a mixing bowl. Line the strainer with cheesecloth or paper towels. Pour the stock through the strainer.

Nutritional Profile

Serving size: 1 cup

Calories: 107
Protein: 6 g
Fiber: 13 g
Fat: 1 g
Saturated fat: 1 g
Sodium: 1,600 mg
Vitamin A: 1,750 IU
Vitamin C: 7 mg

Chicken-Vegetable Noodle Bowls

SERVES 4

People say chicken soup is good for the soul, but it is also good for a healthy serving of lutein, vitamin A, zeaxanthin, and beta-carotene. By adding the broccoli and snow peas sequentially to boiling water, you ensure their tenderness and save on pots to wash.

SAUCE

3 tablespoons low-sodium soy sauce

2 tablespoons rice wine vinegar

2 tablespoons ketchup

2 tablespoons smooth peanut butter

2 tablespoons dark brown sugar

2 tablespoons hoisin sauce

1 teaspoon sriracha hot sauce, or to taste

MARINADE

2 tablespoons low-sodium soy sauce

2 tablespoons rice wine vinegar

1 tablespoon toasted sesame oil

1 tablespoon dark brown sugar

1 pound boneless, skinless chicken breasts or thighs, cut into bite-sized pieces

8 ounces linguine or other noodles

2 cups small broccoli florets

1 cup thinly sliced carrots

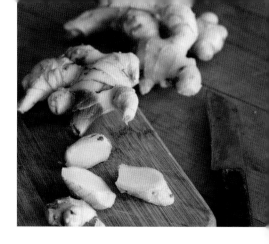

1 cup snow peas

1 tablespoon vegetable or peanut oil

1 small onion, cut into thin wedges

1 tablespoon minced fresh ginger

2 garlic cloves, minced

1 red bell pepper, cut into thin strips

¼ cup chopped cilantro leaves, optional

¼ cup chopped peanuts, optional

In a bowl or blender, combine all the sauce ingredients. Set aside.

Prepare the marinade. In a large bowl, combine the soy sauce, vinegar, sesame oil, and brown sugar. Add the chicken and toss to coat well. Marinate, covered, for 30 to 60 minutes in the refrigerator.

Cook the pasta according to the package directions until al dente (just firm). Add the broccoli and carrots 3 minutes before the pasta is finished. Add the snow peas 1 minute before the pasta is done. Drain well and set aside.

Meanwhile, heat the oil in a large skillet over medium-high heat. Add the onion and ginger and sauté for 3 minutes. Add the garlic and red bell pepper and sauté until fragrant, 1 minute.

Drain the chicken, shaking off and discarding excess marinade, and add it to the pan. Sauté for 3 to 5 minutes, until just cooked through. Add the reserved pasta and vegetables and stir to combine. Add the reserved sauce to the pasta mixture and stir to coat.

Divide among four bowls and sprinkle with the cilantro and peanuts, if using.

Nutritional Profile

Serving size: 1 cup

Calories: 655

Protein: 41 g

Fiber: 6 g

Fat: 22 g

Saturated fat: 4 g

Sodium: 1,323 mg

Vitamin A: 2,819 IU

Vitamin C: 101 mg

Vitamin E: 4 IU

Zinc: 3 mg

Beta-carotene: 631 µg

Lutein and zeaxanthin: 139 µg

Lycopene: 1,253 µg

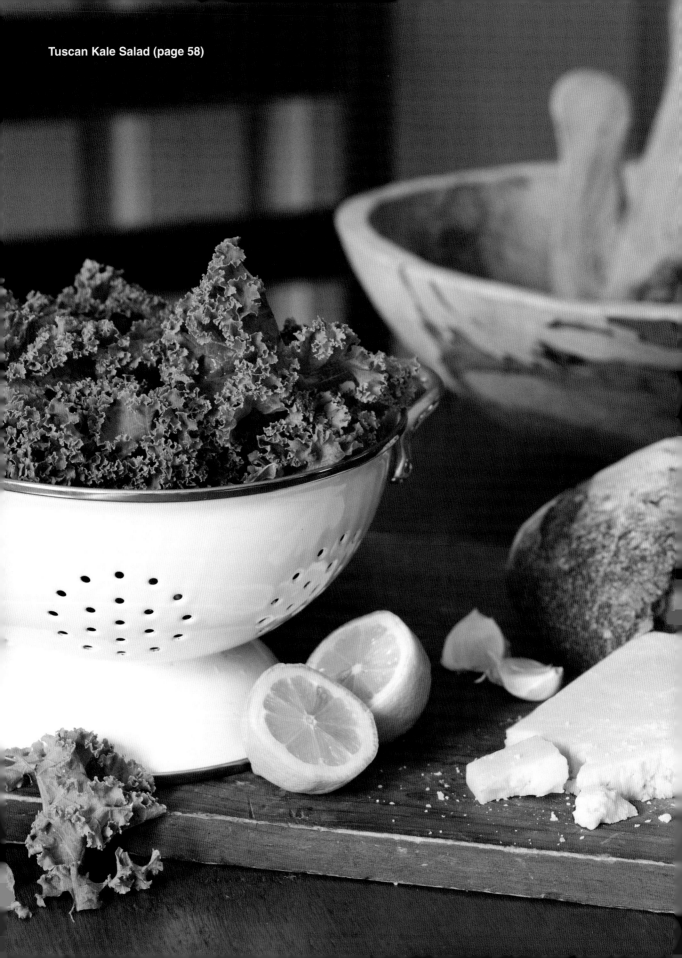

Tuscan Kale Salad (page 58)

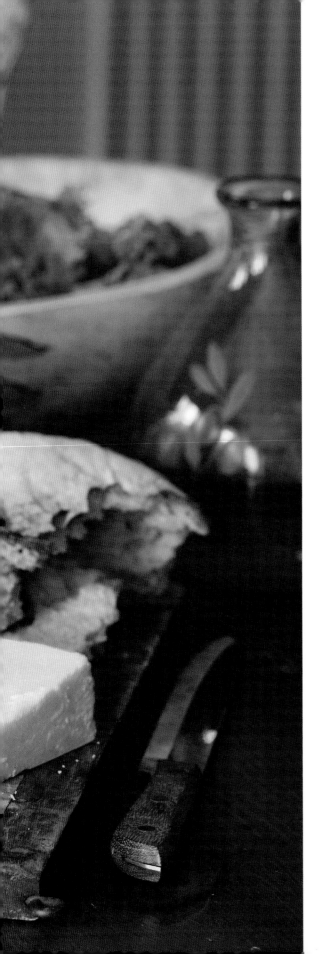

Salads

Tuscan Kale Salad

Celery, Grapefruit, and
  Avocado Salad

Spinach Salad with Walnuts
  and Goji Berries

Spinach Salad with Cured
  Salmon and Poached Egg

Greek Salad

Crunchy Cabbage Salad

Grilled Vegetable Salad

Roasted Butternut Squash
  and Cranberry Salad

Three-Bean Salad

Caprese Salad

Mango Pico de Gallo

Tabbouleh

Toasted Quinoa Salad

Tuscan Kale Salad

One of the most common green vegetables in Europe until the 1400s, raw kale has once again become a star in the garden; with more lutein than other greens, it has powerful antioxidant activity and is rich in beta-carotene, vitamin C, and zeaxanthin. When chopped, kale also releases a chemical called sulforaphane, which is thought to have anti-cancer properties. This recipe is from health guru Dr. Andrew Weil and his True Food Kitchen in Phoenix.

	Juice of 1 lemon
3 to 4	tablespoons extra virgin olive oil
2	garlic cloves, mashed
	Sea salt and freshly ground black pepper to taste
	Red pepper flakes, to taste
4 to 6	cups loosely packed, sliced leaves of Italian black (lacinato, "dinosaur," *cavolo nero*) kale, tough stems removed
⅔	cup grated Pecorino Toscano cheese (Rosselino variety if you can find it) or other flavorful grating cheese such as Asiago or Parmesan
½	cup freshly made bread crumbs from lightly toasted bread

Whisk together the lemon juice, olive oil, garlic, salt, black pepper, and a generous pinch (or more to taste) of the red pepper flakes. Pour over the kale in a serving bowl and toss well. Add two thirds of the cheese and toss again. Let the kale sit for at least 10 minutes. Add the bread crumbs, toss again, and top with the remaining cheese.

Nutritional Profile

Serving size: 1 cup

Calories: 340
Protein: 13 g
Fiber: 3 g
Fat: 21 g
Saturated fat: 5 g
Sodium: 650 mg
Vitamin A: 17,388 IU
Vitamin C: 142 mg
Vitamin E: 3 IU
Zinc: 1 mg
Beta-carotene: 10,349 µg
Lutein and zeaxanthin: 44,188 µg

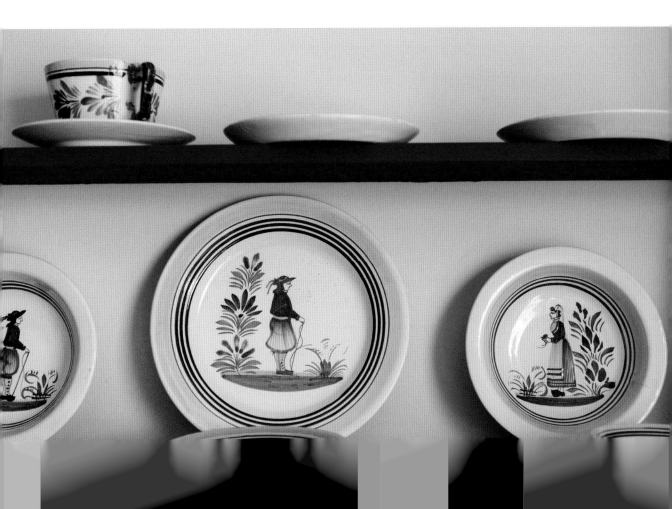

Celery, Grapefruit, and Avocado Salad

SERVES 4–6

This bright salad highlights several preferred ingredients for fighting age-related eye diseases. Pink grapefruit contains lycopene, shown to reduce inflammation and prevent cell damage. When you pair grapefruit with avocado, the avocado's healthy fats help increase lycopene absorption, making it more available for your body to use.

4	pink grapefruits
12	celery ribs
2	avocados
¼	teaspoon ground cumin
2	teaspoons olive oil
1	teaspoon honey
	Sea salt
¼	cup freshly chopped parsley, for garnish

Prepare the grapefruits according to the instructions on page 49.

Using a sharp knife, slice the celery thinly on a deep angle to create elongated Vs. Place in a serving bowl. Top with the grapefruit slices (reserve the juice). Cut each avocado lengthwise in half. Remove and discard the pit. Use a large spoon to scoop the fruit out of the shell in 1 piece. Cut crosswise into half-moon slices. Place on top of the grapefruit slices.

CONTINUED

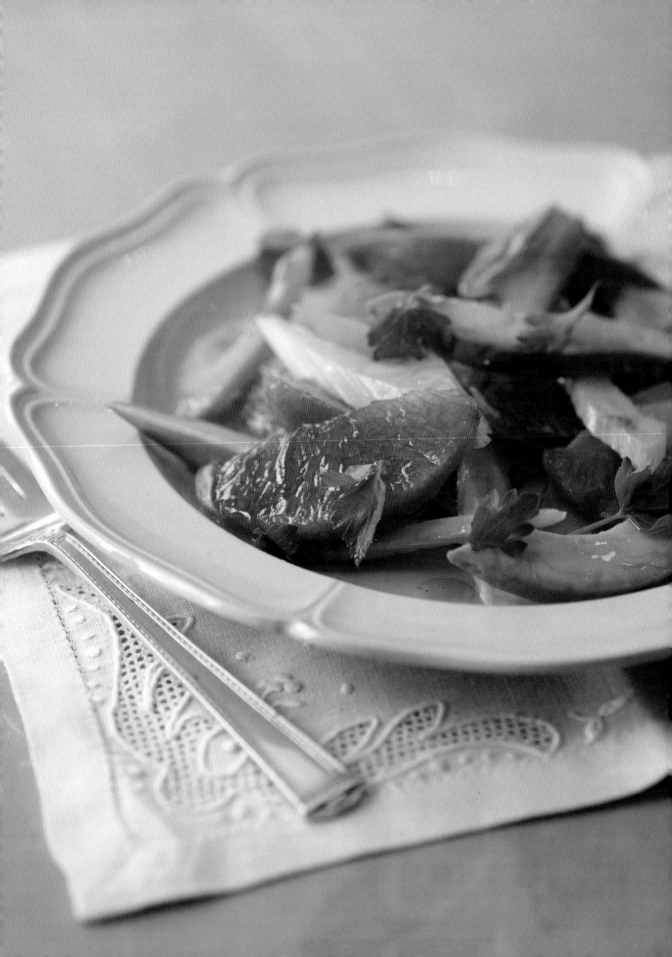

Place the cumin in a dry skillet over medium-high heat. Gently stir or shake the pan. When it becomes fragrant, add the olive oil and honey; swirl to combine. Remove from the heat. Add 2 tablespoons of the reserved grapefruit juice and a generous pinch of salt; swirl to combine. Pour over the salad. Garnish with the parsley. Gently toss at the table.

Nutritional Profile

Serving size: 1 cup

Calories: 200

Protein: 3 g

Fiber: 8 g

Fat: 14 g

Saturated fat: 2 g

Sodium: 220 mg

Vitamin A: 1,754 IU

Vitamin C: 50 mg

Vitamin E: 3 IU

Zinc: 1 mg

Beta-carotene: 1,028 µg

Lutein and zeaxanthin: 665 µg

Lycopene: 1,162 µg

Tip: If not serving immediately, prepare the dressing and set it aside. Brush the avocado slices with some of the reserved grapefruit juice, cover the salad with plastic wrap, and store in the refrigerator for up to 2 hours.

"Why not go out on a limb? Isn't that where the fruit is?"

— *Frank Scully, author*

Good Food Combos

Sometimes the sum is more than the parts, especially in food. Try these combinations when putting together a meal:

Iron and vitamin C: Vitamin C enhances the absorption of the iron found in plant foods. Particularly for vegetarians or individuals who eat small amounts of animal foods, pairing an excellent vitamin C source with a great iron source is beneficial. To increase the iron from a spinach salad, sprinkle it with lemon juice or add orange sections, strawberry slices, or tomatoes. When eating lentils, add vitamin C–rich red bell pepper slices.

Vitamin D and calcium: Vitamin D—the "sunshine vitamin"—is needed for calcium to be absorbed. In the cloudy Pacific Northwest and other northern regions, our bodies are unable to make vitamin D for most of the year. There are few food sources of vitamin D, so many people require a supplement to maintain healthy levels. Examples of foods that do contain vitamin D and calcium include fortified milk and canned salmon.

Vitamins A, D, E, and K: All of these vitamins are fat soluble, so the presence of dietary fat helps with their absorption. Just a small amount of fat is needed, such as a drizzle of olive oil. Avocados and nuts contain their own source of fat along with their own fat-soluble vitamins. Good combinations are avocado with grapefruit, salad dressing with greens, and broccoli rabe with pine nuts.

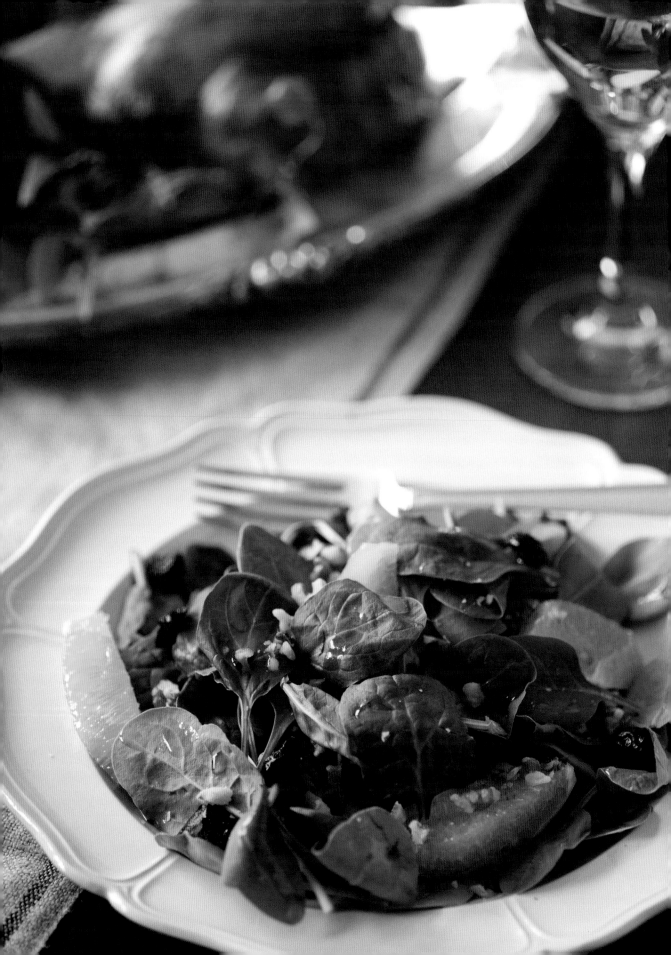

Spinach Salad with Walnuts and Goji Berries

SERVES 4–6

This salad is packed with nutrition—baby spinach provides lutein and zeaxanthin, wheat germ lends vitamin E, walnuts offer vitamin E and zinc, oranges have vitamin C (helping you absorb the spinach's iron), and goji berries contain zeaxanthin, a carotenoid. Toasting the walnuts releases the oils and intensifies the flavor; leaving them raw will maximize the potential health benefits. Goji berries are a nutritionally rich superfruit from a shrub native to China. They can be found in health food and gourmet markets.

- ½ cup extra virgin olive oil
- ¼ cup balsamic vinegar
  - Pinch of sea salt
  - Freshly ground black pepper
- 6 cups baby spinach
- ½ cup finely chopped walnuts
- ⅓ cup dried goji berries (or substitute cranberries)
- 2 tablespoons wheat germ
- 2 segmented navel oranges
  - (see Preparing Citrus Fruit, page 49)

Nutritional Profile

Serving size: 1 cup

Calories: 366
Protein: 4 g
Fiber: 4 g
Fat: 31 g
Saturated fat: 4 g
Sodium: 121 mg
Vitamin A: 1,170 IU
Vitamin C: 37 mg
Vitamin E: 5 IU
Zinc: 1 mg
Beta-carotene: 661 µg
Lutein and zeaxanthin: 1,595 µg
Omega-3 fatty acids: 1 g

In a small bowl, whisk together the olive oil and balsamic vinegar. Season with salt and pepper and set aside. In a salad bowl, combine the spinach, walnuts, goji berries, and wheat germ. Toss with the vinaigrette. Add the orange segments. Season to taste and serve.

Spinach Salad with Cured Salmon and Poached Egg

SERVES 4

From the beloved Green Street Café in Northampton, Massachusetts, which locals still miss, this dish has a lot of lutein and zeaxanthin as well as omega-3 fatty acids. Spinach can be found year-round and refrigerates well.

1	teaspoon distilled white vinegar
4	large eggs
16	cups loosely packed baby spinach
4	garlic cloves, finely chopped
1	large red onion, thinly sliced
1	teaspoon sea salt, plus more to taste
¼	teaspoon freshly ground black pepper, plus more to taste
¼	cup balsamic vinegar
½	cup extra virgin olive oil
¼	cup freshly grated Parmesan cheese
16	strips cured salmon (chiffonade)

To poach the eggs, fill a large bowl with warm water and set it aside. Fill a large skillet with 2 inches of water, add the white vinegar, and bring it to a boil over medium-high heat. Break one of the eggs into a ramekin or teacup. Using the handle (not the bowl) of a wooden spoon, swirl the water in the pot to create a whirlpool, which will help the eggs hold their shape.

CONTINUED

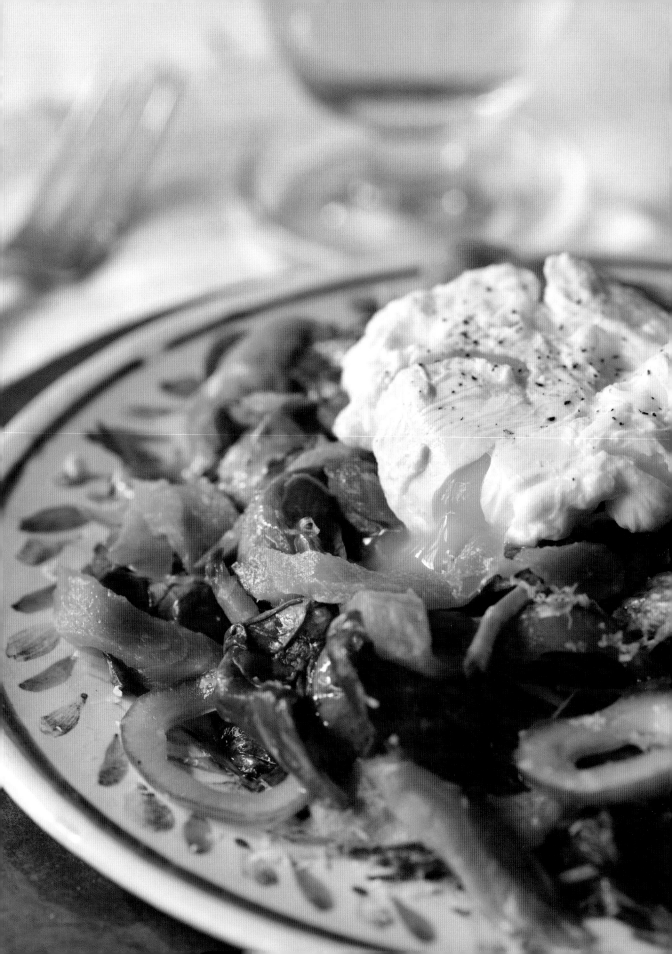

Decrease the heat to medium-low so the water is at a gentle boil, and slide an egg into the center. Adjust the heat, if necessary, to keep the water at a bare simmer and repeat for each egg, poaching until the white is solid and the yolk is firm but soft to the touch, 3 to 4 minutes. (Depending on the pot size, you may need to work in batches.) Transfer with a slotted spoon to the bowl of warm water.

Heat a large sauté pan over medium heat.

Pile the spinach in a metal bowl, then add the garlic and red onion on top of it. Season with salt and pepper and pour the balsamic vinegar on top. When the sauté pan is hot, pour the olive oil into the pan, wait until the oil is smoking, and then add the spinach mixture. Cook until just wilted.

Divide the spinach evenly among four plates and sprinkle each with Parmesan cheese and cured salmon. Pat the eggs dry with a paper towel and place atop the salad. Season to taste with salt and pepper. Serve immediately.

Nutritional Profile

Serving size: 1 cup

Calories: 533
Protein: 35 g
Fiber: 3 g
Fat: 38 g
Saturated fat: 6 g
Sodium: 1,133 mg
Vitamin A: 11,342 IU
Vitamin C: 37 mg
Vitamin D: 1 IU
Vitamin E: 9 IU
Zinc: 2 mg
Beta-carotene: 6,756 µg
Lutein and zeaxanthin: 14,641 µg
Omega-3 fatty acids: 3 g

Greek Salad

SERVES 4–6

There is a potential link between eating a lot of tomatoes and reducing your risk of age-related diseases, including heart disease and cancer. While the studies aren't conclusive, tomatoes—which are high in vitamin A, vitamin C, calcium, folate, potassium, and lycopene—may help promote vibrant health, including healthy eyes.

20	cherry tomatoes, halved
2	cucumbers, peeled, halved, and sliced ½ inch thick
½	small red onion, thinly sliced
3	ounces feta cheese, diced
15	kalamata olives, pitted and quartered
¼	cup extra virgin olive oil
2	tablespoons red wine vinegar
2	teaspoons freshly chopped oregano
	Freshly ground black pepper

In a bowl, toss the ingredients gently to blend. Let them sit for 10 minutes before serving.

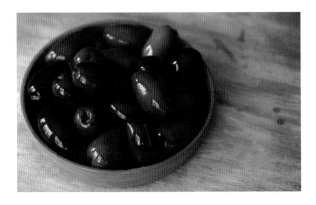

Nutritional Profile

Serving size: 1 cup

Calories: 199
Protein: 5 g
Fiber: 2 g
Fat: 17 g
Saturated fat: 4 g
Sodium: 400 mg
Vitamin A: 787 IU
Vitamin C: 13 mg
Vitamin E: 3 IU
Beta-carotene: 348 µg
Lutein and zeaxanthin: 116 µg
Lycopene: 1,750 µg

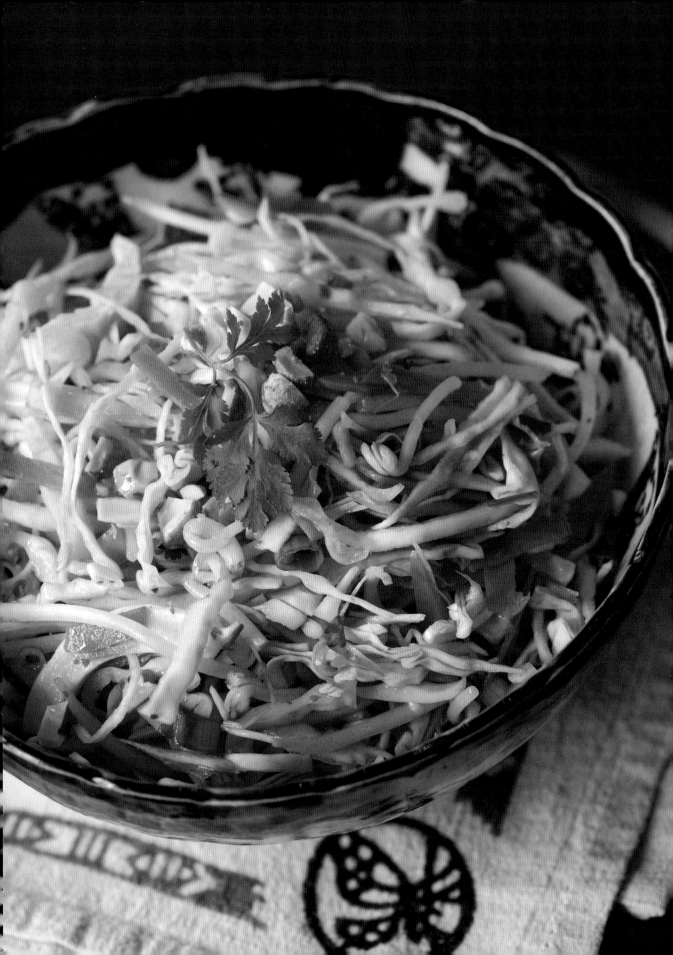

Crunchy Cabbage Salad

SERVES 4–6

This Vietnamese salad has a little kick; to tone down the heat, use less chili garlic sauce. Make a meal of it by serving with sliced, grilled chicken breast. Lutein is abundant in greens, cabbage included, so you may be doing your eyes a favor.

2   teaspoons red chili garlic sauce

⅓   cup rice wine vinegar

2   teaspoons soy sauce

1   tablespoon minced fresh ginger

¼   teaspoon minced garlic

3   tablespoons sesame oil

6   cups shredded green cabbage

2   carrots, chopped or julienned

3   tablespoons freshly shredded cilantro leaves, plus more for garnish

¾   cup bean sprouts

1   small red onion, chopped

¼   cup roasted peanuts, finely chopped

Whisk the first five ingredients in a large bowl, then slowly whisk in the oil. Add the cabbage, carrots, cilantro, bean sprouts, and red onion. Toss and marinate for an hour or more. Garnish with the peanuts and cilantro when ready to serve.

Nutritional Profile

Serving size: 1 cup

Calories: 215
Protein: 6 g
Fiber: 5 g
Fat: 14 g
Saturated fat: 2 g
Sodium: 219 mg
Vitamin A: 5,215 IU
Vitamin C: 41 mg
Vitamin E: 2 IU
Zinc: 1 mg
Beta-carotene: 2,609 µg
Lutein and zeaxanthin: 448 µg

Grilled Vegetable Salad

SERVES 4–6

With salads, don't be tempted to forgo the dressing; recent research has shown that the oil helps you access the nutrients in the vegetables. You might also toss this grilled vegetable dish with greens such as lettuce, arugula, and cilantro for a light supper. Add lentils, grilled fresh salmon, or canned salmon (with bones) for a heartier salad.

- 4 medium tomatoes, cored and halved
- 2 medium zucchini, cut lengthwise into 3 slices
- 2 medium yellow squash, cut lengthwise into 3 slices
- 1 large red bell pepper, cored, seeded, and quartered
- 1 large yellow bell pepper, cored, seeded, and quartered
- 1 medium red onion, sliced ½ inch thick
- 2 portobello mushrooms, sliced ½ inch thick
- 2 tablespoons olive oil
- 1 tablespoon capers, drained
- ½ teaspoon coarse salt

VINAIGRETTE

- 2 tablespoons champagne vinegar
- 6 tablespoons olive oil
- 2 tablespoons fresh basil, cut into thin strips
- 1 garlic clove, minced
- 1 teaspoon fine sea salt
- ½ teaspoon freshly ground black pepper

Preheat the grill to medium-high. Combine the vegetables in a large bowl and toss to coat with the olive oil, capers, and salt.

Grill the vegetables until tender, 5 to 8 minutes on each side, removing them as they become tender. Let them cool.

Cut the cooked, cooled vegetables into bite-sized pieces and combine in a bowl.

To prepare the vinaigrette: Whisk the ingredients together in a small bowl. Toss gently with the vegetables. Season to taste. Serve warm or chilled.

Nutritional Profile

Serving size: 1 cup

Calories: 290

Protein: 5 g

Fiber: 4 g

Fat: 23 g

Saturated fat: 3 g

Sodium: 725 mg

Vitamin A: 1,555 IU

Vitamin C: 160 mg

Vitamin E: 6 IU

Zinc: 1 mg

Beta-carotene: 848 µg

Lutein and zeaxanthin: 3,420 µg

Lycopene: 190 µg

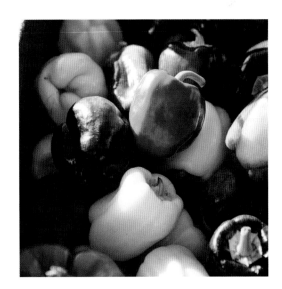

Roasted Butternut Squash and Cranberry Salad

SERVES 4–6

A good source of carotenoids, vitamins A, B6, C, and folate, butternut squash is also rich in phytochemicals, which convert into antioxidants, thought not only to help prevent macular degeneration, but also to reduce the risk for certain cancers and cardiovascular problems. This is a pretty salad that offers a colorful change of pace with its roasted squash, goat cheese, pecans, and cranberries.

1	small butternut squash, peeled, seeded, and cut into ½-inch chunks (about 2 cups)
½	cup extra virgin olive oil
2	tablespoons agave nectar
1¼	teaspoons sea salt
1	teaspoon freshly ground black pepper
One	5-ounce bag baby greens
¼	cup dried cranberries
¼	cup pecan halves, lightly chopped
¼	cup crumbled goat cheese
3	tablespoons white wine vinegar
2	teaspoons whole grain Dijon mustard
1	tablespoon freshly snipped chives

CONTINUED

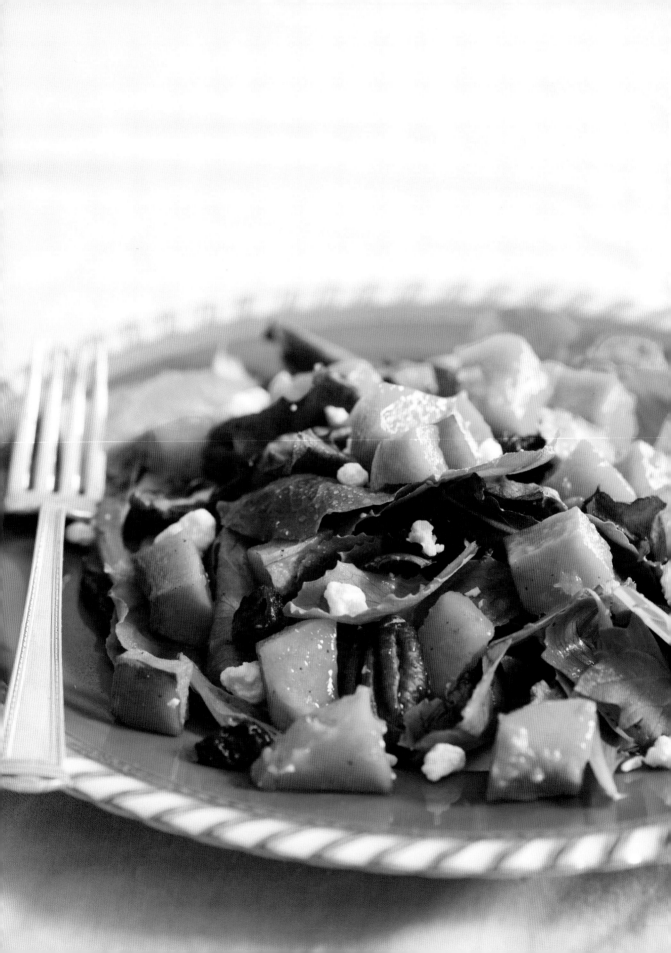

Preheat the oven to 350°F. In a mixing bowl, toss the butternut squash with 2 tablespoons of olive oil, the agave nectar, and 1 teaspoon each of the salt and pepper. Spread in a single layer on a rimmed baking sheet lined with parchment. Bake until tender and golden, 20 to 25 minutes, tossing after 10 minutes. Set aside to cool.

Assemble the baby greens, cranberries, pecans, and goat cheese in a salad bowl. Top with the butternut squash. In a small bowl, whisk together the remaining olive oil, vinegar, mustard, chives, ¼ teaspoon salt, and extra pepper into a vinaigrette and toss with the salad. Serve immediately.

Nutritional Profile

Serving size: 1 cup

Calories: 360
Protein: 4 g
Fiber: 4 g
Fat: 30 g
Saturated fat: 5 g
Sodium: 260 mg
Vitamin A: 10,343 IU
Vitamin C: 6 mg
Vitamin D: 3 IU
Vitamin E: 13 IU
Zinc: 1 mg
Beta-carotene: 3,774 µg
Lutein and zeaxanthin: 5,000 µg

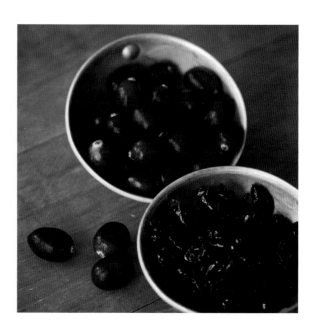

Three-Bean Salad

SERVES 6

Quick to assemble, this salad lends itself to "mix and match" ingredients—if you don't have one type of bean, substitute another. The goal is a blend of flavors and textures. For added crunch, substitute 1½ cups of cut fresh green beans for one of the cans of beans. Black beans are high in protein, folate, iron, magnesium, and potassium, all excellent for eye health. Kidney beans share these benefits and are also rich in vitamin C and niacin. Chickpeas, also known as garbanzos, provide zinc and folate. Some stores carry canned beans that are salt-free.

One   15-ounce can black beans, butter beans, or cannellini beans

One   15-ounce can red beans, such as kidney or adzuki

One   15-ounce can chickpeas

½   cup extra virgin olive oil

¼   cup white wine vinegar

2   garlic cloves, minced

Sea salt

Freshly ground black pepper

1   teaspoon freshly chopped cilantro, or to taste

1   red bell pepper, cored, seeded, and diced

½   red onion, very thinly sliced

Nutritional Profile

Serving size: 1 cup

Calories: 350
Protein: 10 g
Fiber: 10 g
Fat: 20 g
Saturated fat: 3 g
Sodium: 490 mg
Vitamin A: 622 IU
Vitamin C: 28 mg
Vitamin E: 4 IU
Beta-carotene: 323 µg
Lutein and zeaxanthin: 11 µg

Rinse and drain the beans in a colander. Set them aside. In a bowl, whisk together the olive oil, vinegar, garlic, salt, and black pepper. Add the cilantro, rinsed beans, red bell pepper, and onion and toss gently to combine. (If you have time, cover and refrigerate the salad for a few hours to allow the flavors to meld.) Bring to room temperature before serving. Season to taste.

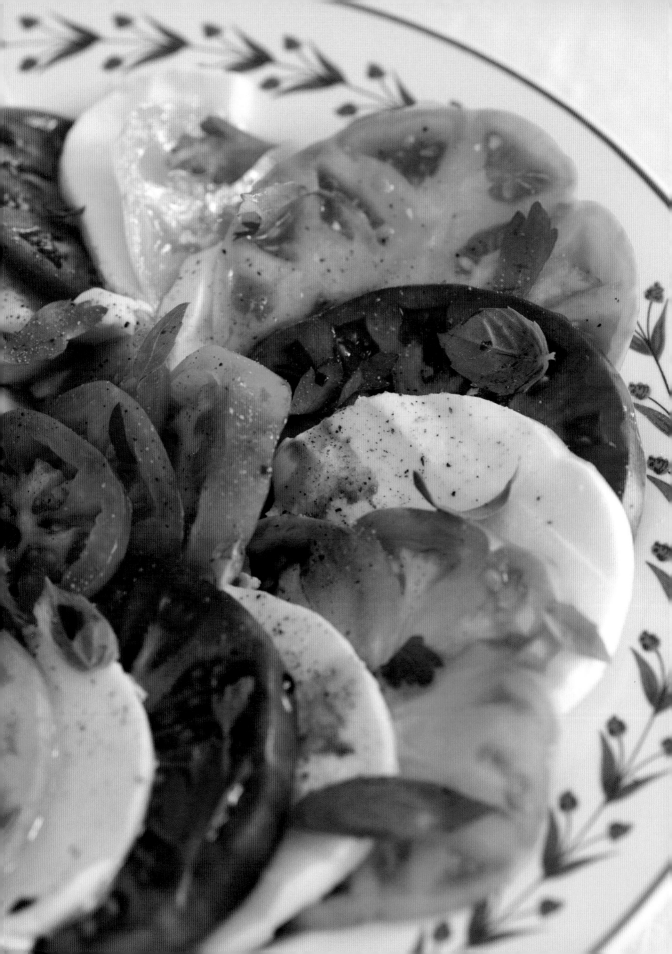

Caprese Salad

L iterally, "a salad from Capri," this dish pairs tomatoes and olive oil, a marriage that helps the body utilize nutrients. Red foods (like tomatoes and watermelon) contain lycopene, an antioxidant that when combined with unsaturated fats is absorbed by the body more readily.

2   Roma tomatoes, cored and sliced

2   yellow tomatoes, cored and sliced

8   ounces fresh mozzarella, thinly sliced

2   tablespoons freshly chopped parsley

2   tablespoons freshly chopped basil

3   tablespoons extra virgin olive oil

1   tablespoon balsamic vinegar

1   garlic clove, minced

    Sea salt

    Freshly ground black pepper

Layer the tomatoes and mozzarella in overlapping fashion, making a circular pattern on a plate. Sprinkle with herbs. In a small bowl, whisk together the olive oil, vinegar, and garlic, then drizzle over the tomatoes. Season to taste with salt and pepper. Serve immediately.

Nutritional Profile

Serving size: 1 cup

Calories: 304

Protein: 16 g

Fiber: 1 g

Fat: 23 g

Saturated fat: 9 g

Sodium: 588 mg

Vitamin A: 692 IU

Vitamin C: 17 mg

Vitamin E: 2 IU

Beta-carotene: 277 µg

Lutein and zeaxanthin: 219 µg

Lycopene: 798 µg

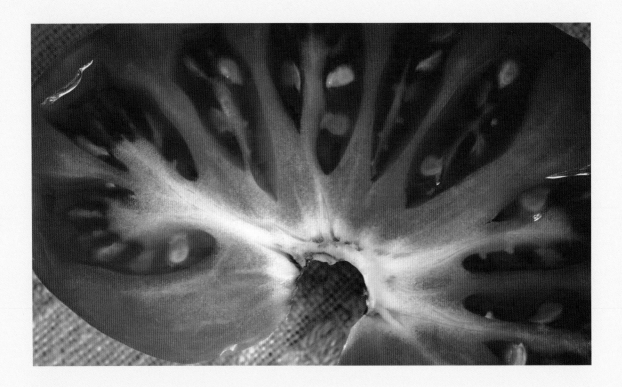

The Amazing Tomato

When introduced to Europe from their native Peru, tomatoes were thought to be poisonous and were enjoyed merely as decoration. Thomas Jefferson was one of the first Americans to serve tomatoes at the table, and in 1820, Robert JoÚson made news when he dared eat one in public. Several ladies fainted, but he didn't die and the tomato took hold in the kitchen. In 1883, when Congress passed a 10 percent tax on imported vegetables, the tomato was called a vegetable to yield more taxes. One importer took the case to the Supreme Court, arguing that it was a berry fruit. He lost the case, and since then the tomato has been classified as a vegetable, although a popular trivia question is to ask whether the tomato is a vegetable or a fruit.

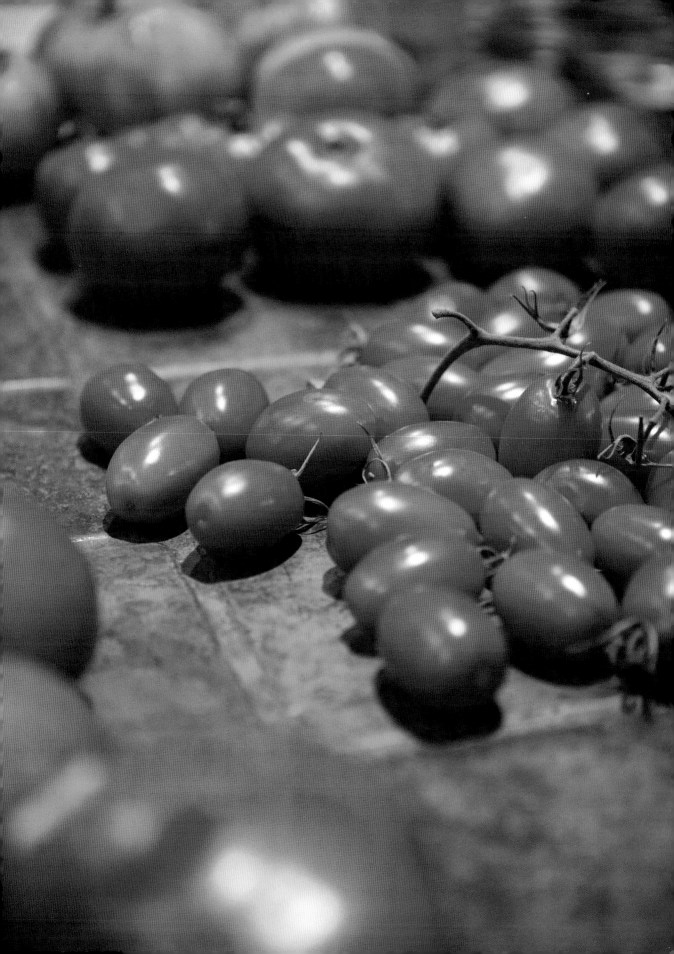

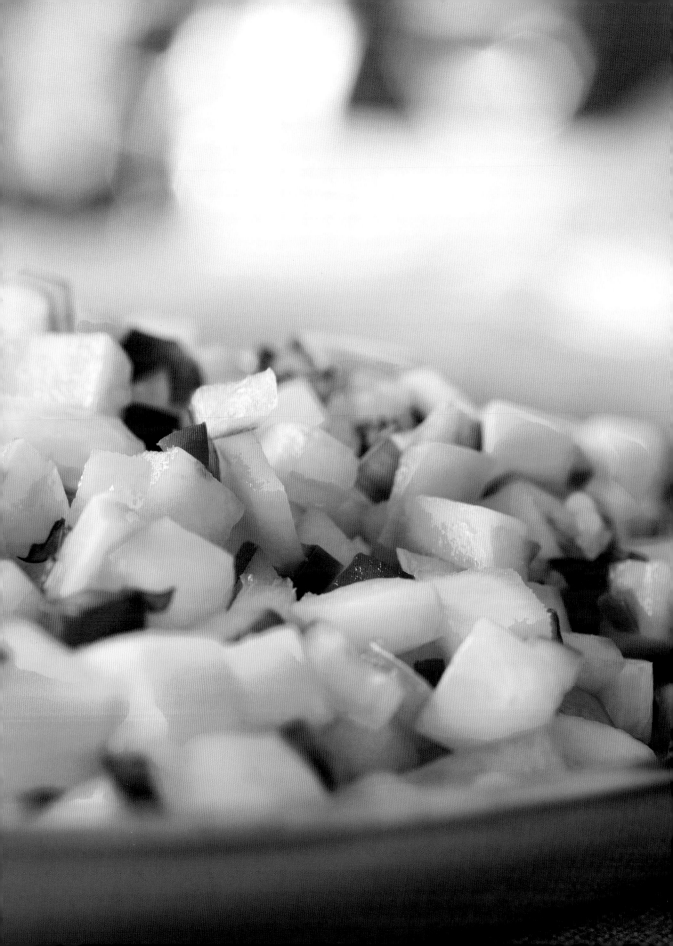

Mango Pico de Gallo

SERVES 4

With its clean, sharp flavors, this dish makes a pretty first course or side dish to fish tacos. A good rule of thumb with eye health is to eat colorful vegetables and fruits every day, since they are high in lutein and zeaxanthin.

- 2 mangoes, peeled, seeded, and diced (about 2 cups)
- 1 small red onion, finely diced
- 2 tablespoons freshly squeezed lime juice
- 1 garlic clove, minced
- 2 cucumbers, peeled, seeded, and diced
- ½ jalapeño, cored, seeded, and diced
- 2 tablespoons diced yellow or red bell pepper
- 2 tablespoons freshly shredded mint leaves

Sea salt

Freshly ground black pepper

Combine all the ingredients in a large bowl. Cover and refrigerate until ready to serve.

Nutritional Profile

Serving size: 1 cup

Calories: 85

Protein: 2 g

Fiber: 3 g

Fat: 1 g

Saturated fat: less than 1 g

Sodium: 157 mg

Vitamin A: 1,279 IU

Vitamin C: 48 mg

Vitamin E: 1 IU

Beta-carotene: 731 µg

Lutein and zeaxanthin: 60 µg

Lycopene: 3 µg

Tabbouleh

SERVES 4–6

A Middle Eastern salad made with couscous or bulgur, tabbouleh is a healthy base to which you can add vegetables that promote eye health. This version uses buckwheat groats, a gluten-free grain also known as kasha. Serve as a side dish or as an appetizer with grape leaves for scooping, as they do in the Middle East. This is a flexible salad; experiment with vegetables and taste as you prepare.

1 cup whole buckwheat groats

1 teaspoon sea salt

½ teaspoon freshly ground black pepper

1 cup freshly chopped parsley

2 tablespoons freshly chopped mint

½ medium red onion, diced

1 medium tomato, cored and diced

1 cucumber, peeled, seeded and diced

6 tablespoons freshly squeezed lemon juice

6 tablespoons extra virgin olive oil

Bring 1 quart (4 cups) of water to a boil in a medium saucepan over high heat. Add the buckwheat and season with salt and pepper. Cook until tender, about 10 minutes. Drain and rinse under cold running water. Place the cooked buckwheat in a bowl. Add the remaining ingredients. Toss gently and serve, or chill until serving.

Nutritional Profile

Serving size: 1 cup

Calories: 304

Protein: 6 g

Fiber: 4 g

Fat: 18 g

Saturated fat: 2 g

Sodium: 587 mg

Vitamin A: 1,196 IU

Vitamin C: 31 mg

Vitamin E: 2 IU

Beta-carotene: 710 µg

Lutein and zeaxanthin: 692 µg

Lycopene: 47 µg

Toasted Quinoa Salad

SERVES 4

Held sacred by the Incas, quinoa is rich in protein and fiber and a low-cholesterol source of complex carbs, providing plant-derived calcium. Quinoa is a seed, rather than a grain. When it cooks, the germ ring (the part of the seed that separates during germination) pops open. Toasting the quinoa yields a nuttier flavor.

1	cup dry quinoa
½	cup freshly chopped chives
¼	cup freshly chopped parsley
2	tablespoons freshly chopped cilantro
1	teaspoon fresh lemon zest
½	teaspoon sea salt
	Freshly ground black pepper

Preheat the oven to 350°F. Rinse the quinoa thoroughly in a mesh strainer. Lightly coat a baking sheet with nonstick cooking spray. Spread the quinoa evenly on the sheet and toast for 10 minutes, stirring after 2 to 3 minutes for even toasting.

Bring 3½ cups of water to a boil in a medium saucepan. Add toasted quinoa. Cook until tender and the germ ring pops open (it will look like a white spiral), about 15 minutes. Drain and cool. Toss the quinoa with the chives, parsley, cilantro, and lemon zest. Season to taste with salt and pepper. Serve immediately.

Nutritional Profile

Serving size: 1 cup

Calories: 160
Protein: 6 g
Fiber: 3 g
Fat: 3 g
Saturated fat: less than 1 g
Sodium: 362 mg
Vitamin A: 592 IU
Vitamin C: 9 mg
Vitamin E: 2 IU
Zinc: 1 mg
Beta-carotene: 355 µg
Lutein and zeaxanthin: 301 µg

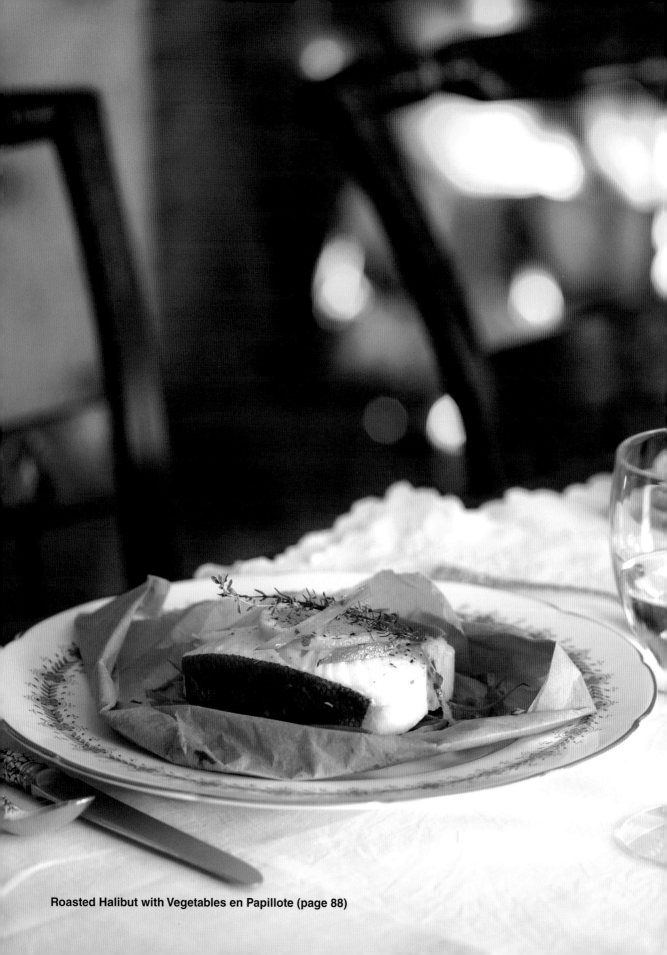

Roasted Halibut with Vegetables en Papillote (page 88)

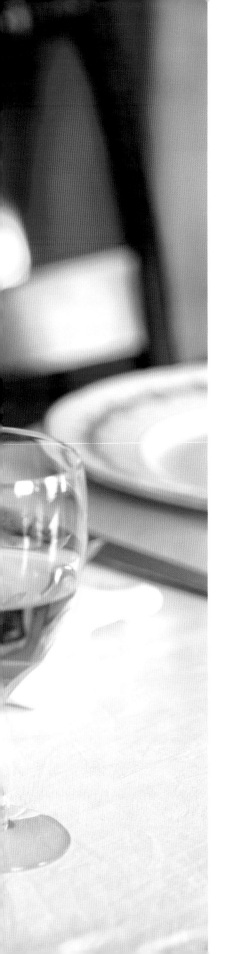

Main Courses

Roasted Halibut with Vegetables en Papillote

Salmon with Peppered Balsamic Strawberries

Grilled Herbed Tuna on Spinach Salad

Spicy Fish Tacos

Grilled Sardines

Sardine Sandwiches

Cornish Game Hens Stuffed with Wild Rice

Chicken with Mushrooms and Thyme

Spinach Omelet

Rice Paper Salmon with Satay Drizzle

Pigs in a Blanket

Garlic-Lime Pork Chops

Stuffed Cabbage

Mini Meatloaves

Pumpkin Pappardelle

Macaroni and Cheese

Red Curry Vegetables with Coconut Sauce

Spicy Udon Noodles

Jacques Pépin's Provence Pizza

Roasted Halibut with Vegetables en Papillote

SERVES 4

Halibut is a good source of vitamin A and protein and is low in fat. *En papillote* means the dish is baked in parchment paper pouches, which can be assembled several hours ahead and refrigerated until ready to bake.

- 4   halibut fillets (about 1½ pounds)
- 4   teaspoons white wine
- 4   teaspoons olive oil
- 1   cup julienned carrots
- 1½ cups julienned snow peas
- ½   red onion, thinly sliced
- ¼   cup freshly chopped parsley
-     Sea salt
-     Freshly ground black pepper
- 4   lemon slices
- 4   sprigs fresh thyme

Preheat the oven to 400°F. Pat the fillets dry. In a medium bowl, combine the white wine, olive oil, carrots, snow peas, and red onion with the parsley, salt, and pepper. Divide the vegetable mixture equally among four 13 by 16-inch sheets of parchment paper, setting them slightly off center. Top each with fish, a lemon slice, and a thyme sprig. Working one packet at a time, fold parchment over the fish to form an envelope. Fold the edges of the parchment into tight ¼-inch folds, creasing each fold securely so the steam won't escape.

Arrange the packets on a baking sheet. Bake until the parchments have puffed and are golden, 10 to 12 minutes. To serve, place the packets on individual plates and cut them open.

Note: To julienne means to cut into matchsticks.

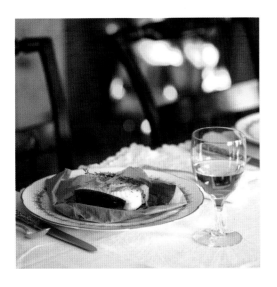

Nutritional Profile

Serving size: 1 fillet

Calories: 310
Protein: 47 g
Fiber: 2 g
Fat: 9 g
Saturated fat: 1 g
Sodium: 323 mg
Vitamin A: 6,197 IU
Vitamin C: 17 mg
Vitamin E: 1 IU
Beta-carotene: 2,917 µg
Lutein and zeaxanthin: 428 µg
Omega-3 fatty acids: .04 g

Salmon with Peppered Balsamic Strawberries

SERVES 4

This recipe from Canyon Ranch, a long-standing health spa, features salmon, which is a good source of omega-3 fatty acids, as well as niacin and magnesium. The lemon and strawberries help with absorption of the iron in the spinach. It's tasty served with ½ cup of Toasted Quinoa Salad (page 85) on the side.

Four	4-ounce salmon fillets
2	teaspoons fresh lemon zest
¼	teaspoon sea salt
¼	teaspoon freshly ground black pepper

PEPPERED BALSAMIC STRAWBERRIES

2	cups small diced fresh strawberries
2	tablespoons fresh basil chiffonade
1	tablespoon balsamic vinegar
1	tablespoon turbinado sugar
½	teaspoon coarsely ground black pepper

½	pound spinach

CONTINUED

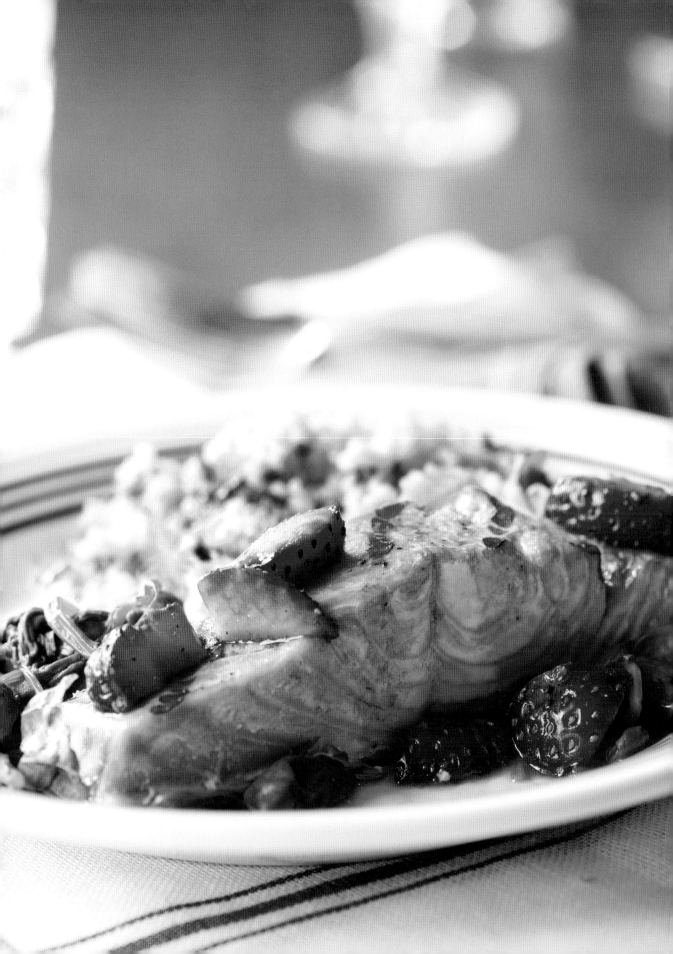

Preheat a grill or broiler. Season the salmon fillets with lemon zest, salt, and pepper. Grill or broil the salmon fillets 3 to 5 minutes on each side, until the fish is cooked through.

In a medium bowl, mix the strawberries, basil, vinegar, sugar, and pepper until well combined.

Steam the spinach to your desired doneness, about 3 to 5 minutes. Evenly divide the steamed spinach among four plates. Place each salmon fillet on greens and top with ½ cup of peppered balsamic strawberries.

Nutritional Profile

Serving size: 1 fillet

Calories: 261
Protein: 31 g
Fiber: 3 g
Fat: 10 g
Saturated fat: 1 g
Sodium: 287 mg
Vitamin A: 5,448 IU
Vitamin C: 62 mg
Vitamin E: 2 IU
Zinc: 1 mg
Beta-carotene: 3,238 µg
Lutein and zeaxanthin: 7,013 µg
Omega-3 fatty acids: 3 g

"The greatest delight the fields and woods minister is the suggestion of an occult relation between man and the vegetable. I am not alone and unacknowledged. They nod to me and I to them."

— *Ralph Waldo Emerson*

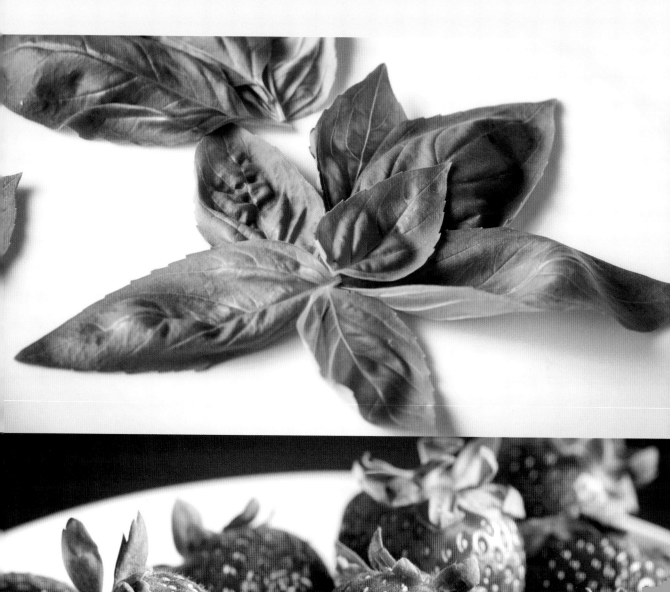

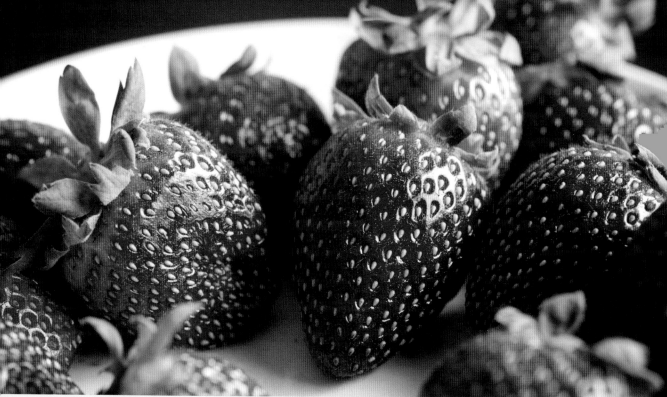

Grilled Herbed Tuna on Spinach Salad

SERVES 6

Seafood contains types of fat called omega-3s that can benefit brain, heart, and eye health. Omega-3s may also reduce depression, relieve joint pain, and boost the immune system, according to some experts. This recipe is from Jacques Pépin.

 2   tablespoons sherry vinegar
 1   small shallot, peeled, trimmed, and chopped (2 tablespoons)
 1   tablespoon chopped fresh tarragon leaves
 ¼   teaspoon freshly ground black pepper
 3   tablespoons extra virgin olive oil
 ¾   teaspoon sea salt
 7   medium button mushrooms (4 ounces), washed and cut into ½ inch dice (1½ cups)
 1   medium tomato, peeled, seeded, and cut into ½-inch pieces (1 cup)
 12 ounces spinach
 1   tablespoon whole black peppercorns, crushed
 1   tablespoon herbes de Provence
 6   center-cut tuna steaks (6 ounces each and about ¾ inch thick)

In a very large bowl, mix the vinegar, shallot, tarragon, ground pepper, 2 tablespoons of the oil, and ¼ teaspoon of the salt. Add the mushrooms and tomato, toss well, and set aside.

Trim, wash, and dry the spinach. Break the leaves into slightly smaller pieces. (You should have about 7 cups.) Set aside.

Pat the crushed pepper and herbes de Provence into the tuna. Sprinkle both sides of the steaks with the remaining tablespoon of oil and the remaining ½ teaspoon of salt.

Preheat a grill until it's very hot.

Arrange the tuna on a clean rack and grill for 1½ minutes on each side for rare (or 2 minutes for medium). Transfer to a large platter and cover with a domed lid.

Add the spinach to the bowl with the dressing mixture; toss well. Divide the salad among six plates.

Cut each tuna steak on the diagonal into 3 pieces and arrange the equivalent of 1 steak on each plate. Serve immediately.

Note: The easiest way to crush whole peppercorns is with the bottom of a heavy pan. Place the peppercorns in a single layer on a flat surface, such as a cutting board. Press down on them with the pan to crack them to the coarseness desired.

Nutritional Profile

Serving size: 1 tuna steak

Calories: 404
Protein: 53 g
Fiber: 2 g
Fat: 18 g
Saturated fat: 4 g
Sodium: 487 mg
Vitamin A: 9,584 IU
Vitamin C: 22 mg
Vitamin D: 1 IU
Vitamin E: 6 IU
Zinc: 2 mg
Beta-carotene: 3,194 µg
Lutein and zeaxanthin: 6,923 µg
Omega-3 fatty acids: 3 g

Spicy Fish Tacos

SERVES 4

A popular roadside snack in Southern California, fish tacos are easy to make and loaded with fiber and nutrients. Top with chopped fresh tomatoes for additional health appeal and color. Feel free to use low-fat mayonnaise and/or yogurt.

½	small red cabbage, shredded (about 2 cups)
½	small green cabbage, shredded (about 2 cups)
¼	cup mayonnaise
¼	cup plain yogurt
1	tablespoon minced chipotle in adobo or chipotle hot sauce
	Juice of ½ lime
¼	cup freshly chopped cilantro
¼	teaspoon sea salt
½	teaspoon freshly ground black pepper
1	pound whitefish, such as cod, halibut, or tilapia fillets
2	tablespoons olive oil
Eight	6-inch flour tortillas
2	cups fresh guacamole (see page 98), for serving
	Hot sauce, for serving
	Lime wedges, for serving

CONTINUED

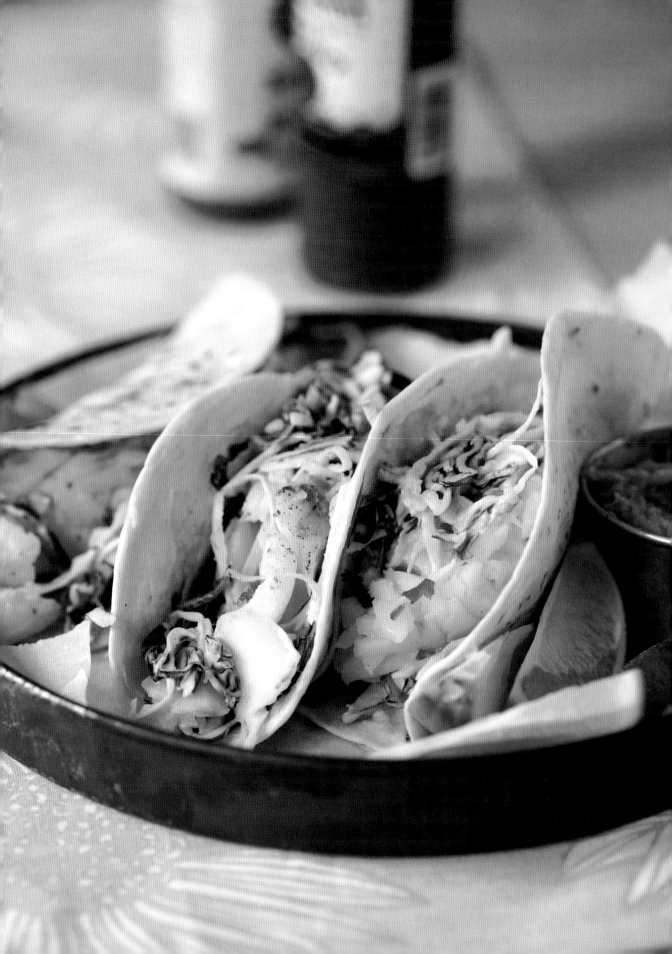

In a large bowl, combine the cabbage with the mayonnaise, yogurt, chipotle in adobo, lime juice, and cilantro. Season with the salt and pepper and set aside.

Season the fish with extra black pepper. Heat the oil in a large nonstick skillet over medium-high heat. Cook the fish 2 to 4 minutes per side or until opaque. Flake the fish with a fork.

Heat the tortillas on a grill or in the oven until pliable, about 20 seconds. Spoon into each tortilla the fish, cabbage mixture, and guacamole. Serve immediately with hot sauce and lime wedges.

Guacamole

MAKES 2 CUPS

- 3 Hass avocados, peeled, pitted, and diced
- 1 small tomato, diced
- ½ small red onion, diced
- 1 garlic clove, minced
- 1 tablespoon extra virgin olive oil
- 1 tablespoon balsamic vinegar
- 1 tablespoon chopped fresh cilantro
  Juice of one fresh lime
- 2 teaspoons hot sauce
  Salt and freshly ground pepper

Blend all ingredients in a bowl. Taste and season more if desired.

Nutritional Profile

Serving size: 2 tacos

Calories: 655
Protein: 40 g
Fiber: 10 g
Fat: 30 g
Saturated fat: 10 g
Sodium: 1,648 mg
Vitamin A: 870 IU
Vitamin C: 92 mg
Vitamin D: 8 IU
Vitamin E: 2 IU
Beta-carotene: 258 µg
Lutein and zeaxanthin: 134 µg
Lycopene: 7 µg
Omega-3 fatty acids: .04 g

Grilled Sardines

SERVES 4

F resh sardines are inexpensive and delicious. Plus, they are nutritional treasures and a refreshing summer meal when served with a Greek Salad (page 69).

¼ cup olive oil

2 garlic cloves, minced

1 tablespoon freshly chopped parsley

4 teaspoons freshly chopped thyme

Sea salt

Freshly ground black pepper

8 medium fresh sardines, gutted

In a bowl, combine the olive oil, garlic, parsley, thyme, salt, and pepper. Add the sardines, stir to coat, and place them in the refrigerator, covered, to marinate for 1 hour.

Heat a grill to medium-high. Remove the sardines from the marinade and grill for 3 to 4 minutes per side, depending on size, until the flesh flakes and the skin is nicely crisped. Brush with the marinade in the first half of the cooking time. Season to taste and serve.

Nutritional Profile

Serving size: 2 sardines

Calories: 214

Protein: 11 g

Fiber: less than 1 g

Fat: 19 g

Saturated fat: 3 g

Sodium: 562 mg

Vitamin A: 148 IU

Vitamin C: 2 mg

Vitamin D: 202 IU

Vitamin E: 4 IU

Zinc: 1 mg

Beta-carotene: 57 µg

Lutein and zeaxanthin: 61 µg

Omega-3 fatty acids: 1 g

Sardine Sandwiches

MAKES 2 SANDWICHES

Small but mighty, sardines have omega-3 fatty acids and vitamin D. Several studies have shown that a diet that includes enough omega-3 fatty acids, including dark-meat fish like sardines, may reduce the risk of developing age-related macular degeneration. Great bread matters with this sandwich.

4 slices hearty whole grain bread

Whole grain Dijon mustard

One 3.75-ounce can of sardines with bones, packed in oil or water, drained

1 medium tomato, cored and sliced

2 scallions, chopped

Freshly ground black pepper

Mayonnaise

Toast the bread. Spread mustard on two slices. Divide the sardines (including bones) evenly and layer them onto the mustard. Add the tomato, scallions, and pepper. Spread mayonnaise on the remaining two slices of bread and close the sandwiches.

Nutritional Profile

Serving size: 1 sandwich

Calories: 390
Protein: 22 g
Fiber: 5 g
Fat: 12 g
Saturated fat: 1 g
Sodium: 886 mg
Vitamin A: 275 IU
Vitamin C: 15 mg
Vitamin D: 103 IU
Vitamin E: 2 IU
Zinc: 1 mg
Beta-carotene: 127 µg
Lutein and zeaxanthin: 184 µg
Lycopene: 118 µg
Omega-3 fatty acids: 1 g

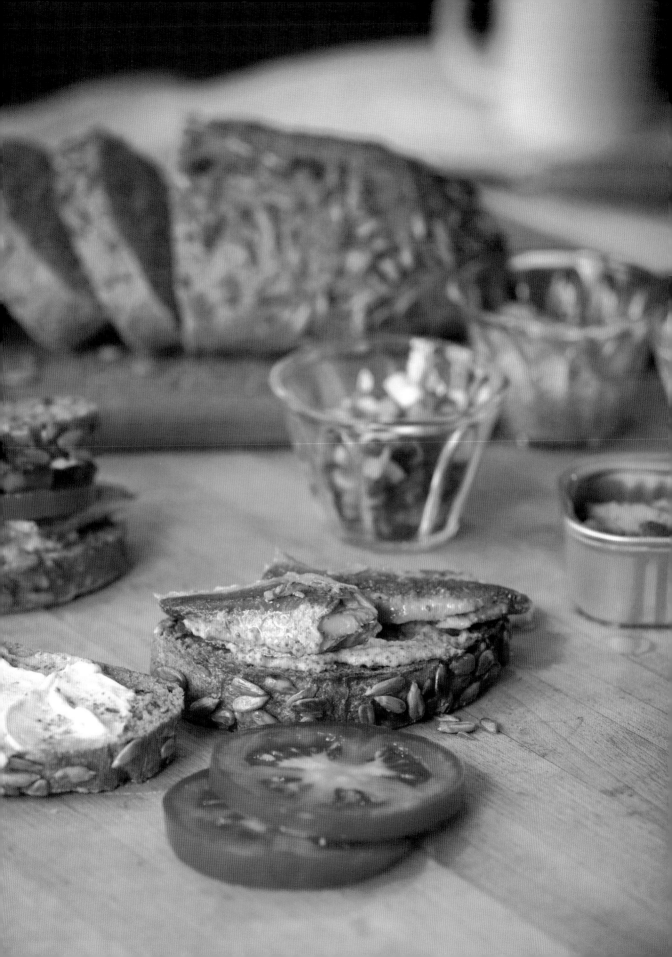

Cornish Game Hens Stuffed with Wild Rice

SERVES 4

Cornish hens are young chickens weighing not more than two pounds. Chicken is a source of lean protein, essential for growth and brain development. The cranberries offer vitamin C and the walnuts provide a dose of omega-3s.

STUFFING

- 2 cups low-sodium chicken stock
- 5 ounces (¾ cup) long-grain wild rice mix
- 2 tablespoons olive oil
- 3 ounces button mushrooms, diced (1 cup)
- 1 tablespoon minced garlic
- 7 scallions, diced small (1 cup)
- ¼ cup dried cranberries
- ¼ cup chopped walnuts
- 1 teaspoon freshly chopped thyme
- ½ teaspoon freshly chopped sage
- ¼ teaspoon sea salt
- ⅛ teaspoon freshly ground black pepper

FOR THE HENS

- 4 Cornish game hens, rinsed and patted dry
- 1 tablespoon plus 1 teaspoon olive oil, divided

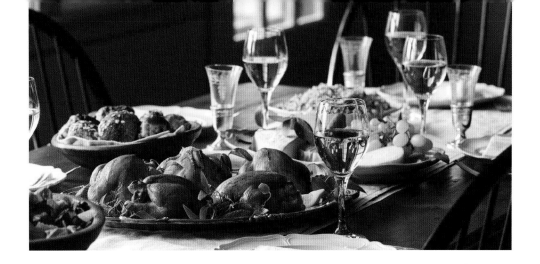

In a medium saucepan, bring the chicken stock to a boil. Add the rice. Cover, reduce the heat to low, and simmer until the rice is tender, about 45 minutes. Remove from the heat and cool.

Meanwhile, heat the olive oil in a medium frying pan over medium-high heat, add the mushrooms, and sauté for 10 minutes. Add the garlic and scallions and sauté for 5 minutes. Remove from the heat and add the cranberries, walnuts, thyme, sage, salt, and pepper. Stir to combine and allow to cool.

Preheat the oven to 350°F. In a medium bowl, combine the rice with the mushroom mixture, stir well, and set aside. Stuff each hen with ¾ cup of the stuffing. Rub 1 teaspoon of olive oil on each hen. Place in an ovenproof dish and bake 1¼ to 1½ hours, until juices run clear. Let it rest 15 minutes, then serve.

Nutritional Profile

Serving size: 1 hen

Calories: 1,026
Protein: 67 g
Fiber: 4 g
Fat: 65 g
Saturated fat: 15 g
Sodium: 1,090 mg
Vitamin A: 708 IU
Vitamin C: 9 mg
Vitamin D: 2 IU
Vitamin E: 4 IU
Zinc: 4 mg
Beta-carotene: 167 µg
Lutein and zeaxanthin: 305 µg
Omega-3 fatty acids: 1 g

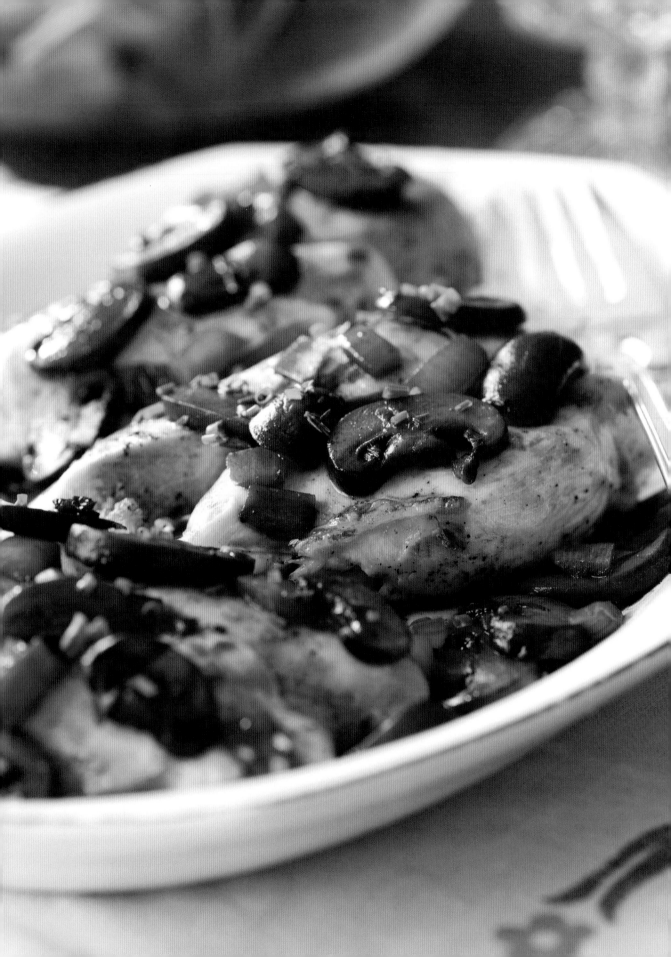

Chicken with Mushrooms and Thyme

SERVES 4

Chicken is dense in niacin, as well as vitamin B—which is good for energy metabolism—and phosphorus, an essential mineral for maintaining healthy teeth and bones.

- 1   tablespoon unsalted butter
- 2   tablespoons olive oil
- 4   boneless, skinless chicken breast halves (about 1½ to 2 pounds)
- ¼   teaspoon sea salt
- ¼   teaspoon freshly ground black pepper
- ⅓   cup chopped yellow onion
- 2   garlic cloves, minced
- 1   cup cremini mushrooms, sliced
- ¼   cup balsamic vinegar
- 1   teaspoon freshly chopped thyme
- 1   tablespoon freshly chopped chives

CONTINUED

Preheat the oven to 350°F. Heat the butter and olive oil over high heat in a heavy saucepan or skillet large enough to hold the chicken breasts in one layer. When the oil smokes, add the chicken breasts and season them with the salt and pepper. Sauté until golden brown, about 3 minutes on each side. Transfer to an oven-safe dish and bake until the juices run clear when pierced with a knife, about 25 minutes. Remove to a plate and keep warm.

Add the onion, garlic, and mushrooms to the drippings in the pan and cook for about 1 minute over high heat. Add the vinegar and thyme and continue cooking for about 1 minute. Add ½ cup of water and cook until the liquid is reduced by half. Season to taste. To serve, slice each breast in half crosswise on the diagonal. Coat the chicken with the sauce and sprinkle with chives.

Nutritional Profile

Serving size: 1 breast

Calories: 314
Protein: 39 g
Fiber: 1 g
Fat: 14 g
Saturated fat: 7 g
Sodium: 388 mg
Vitamin A: 189 IU
Vitamin C: 4 mg
Vitamin D: 12 IU
Vitamin E: 2 IU
Zinc: 1 mg
Beta-carotene: 34 µg
Lutein and zeaxanthin: 10 µg

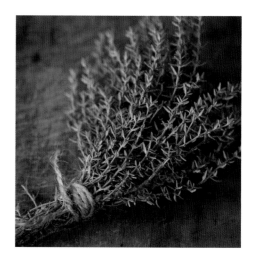

Spinach Omelet

SERVES 1

Cooking the spinach just briefly serves to help your body retain more of its carotenoids, lutein, and zeaxanthin.

- 1 teaspoon olive oil
- 1 tablespoon finely diced yellow onion
- 1 tablespoon finely diced mushrooms
- 1 cup baby spinach, stemmed and chopped
- 2 large eggs
- 1 teaspoon freshly chopped chives
- 1 teaspoon freshly chopped parsley
- Sea salt and freshly ground black pepper
- 1 teaspoon unsalted butter
- 1 teaspoon olive oil
- 2 tablespoons grated low-fat mozzarella cheese

In an 8-inch sauté pan, heat the oil over medium-high heat, then add the onion and mushroom. Cook until softened, about 8 to 10 minutes, then add the spinach and cook for 1 minute. Remove from the heat and place in a bowl.

Break the eggs into a small bowl and beat with the chives, parsley, salt, and pepper.

In the same pan, on medium heat, add the butter and oil, swirling to coat the sides of the pan. When the butter is melted, add the egg, swirling to distribute, and cook until bottom is set, shaking the eggs and lifting the edges with a fork to allow eggs to flow underneath if necessary. Add the cooked vegetables and sprinkle cheese on one side, then fold in half and cook for 1 minute, or until the cheese is melted. Slide it onto a plate and serve.

Nutritional Profile

Serving size: 1 omelet

Calories: 314
Protein: 18 g
Fiber: 2 g
Fat: 25 g
Saturated fat: 8 g
Sodium: 897 mg
Vitamin A: 1,819 IU
Vitamin C: 7 mg
Vitamin D: 85 IU
Vitamin E: 4 IU
Zinc: 1 mg
Beta-carotene: 608 µg
Lutein and zeaxanthin: 1,845 µg

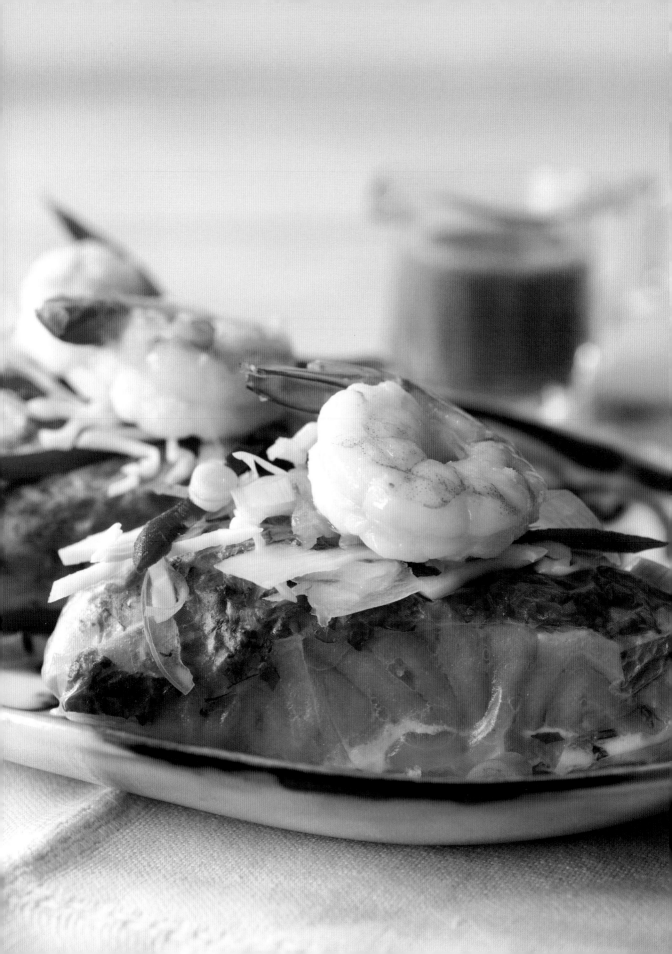

Rice Paper Salmon with Satay Drizzle

SERVES 4

In this globally inspired recipe from the Lake Austin Spa Resort, the rice paper is used in a fashion similar to the French technique of baking in parchment (en papillote), which keeps the food moist and flavorful—but rice paper is edible. The sheets come in varying shapes and sizes. You should prepare the Satay Sauce (next page) first.

Four 12-inch round rice paper sheets (found in gourmet grocery stores or Asian markets)

2 tablespoons freshly chopped mint leaves

2 tablespoons freshly chopped basil leaves

2 tablespoons freshly chopped cilantro leaves

Four 3-ounce skinless salmon fillets

Sea salt and freshly ground black pepper

½ small green cabbage, shredded (about 2 cups)

1 cup very thinly sliced red, yellow, and/or green bell peppers

6 scallions, sliced

1 jalapeño, cored, seeded, and thinly sliced

8 slices (2 tablespoons) pink pickled ginger

4 large cooked shrimp, peeled, deveined, and chilled (optional)

CONTINUED

Submerge 1 sheet of rice paper in a large bowl of very hot tap water for 15 seconds, or until it is completely pliant. Remove it from the water and spread it on a clean flat surface. Sprinkle one quarter of the mint, basil, and cilantro over the surface. Arrange 1 salmon fillet in the center. Season the salmon with salt and pepper. Fold one side of the rice paper over the fish, then fold in the remaining sides. Continue to roll and encase the salmon. Repeat the process with the remaining sheets.

Preheat the oven to 400°F. Spray a baking sheet lightly with nonstick cooking spray. Arrange the salmon packages, seam side down, not touching each other, on the baking sheet. Bake for 12 to 15 minutes. Toss the cabbage, bell peppers, scallions, and jalapeño in a bowl. Arrange 1 salmon package in the center of each of four plates. Top with slaw, 2 slices of pickled ginger, and 1 shrimp, if using. Drizzle Satay Sauce over the top.

Satay Sauce

¼ cup reduced-fat smooth all-natural peanut butter

Grated zest and juice of 1 lime

2 tablespoons brown sugar

2 tablespoons light soy sauce

1 tablespoon minced fresh ginger

1 garlic clove, minced

2 teaspoons Asian chili paste

2 teaspoons pure coconut extract

Combine the peanut butter, ⅓ cup of hot water, lime zest and juice, brown sugar, soy sauce, ginger, garlic, chili paste, and coconut extract in a bowl, mix well, and set aside.

Nutritional Profile

Serving size: 1 fillet

Calories: 387

Protein: 31 g

Fiber: 4 g

Fat: 16 g

Saturated fat: 4 g

Sodium: 723 mg

Vitamin A: 1,322 IU

Vitamin C: 60 mg

Vitamin D: 2 IU

Vitamin E: 3 IU

Zinc: 2 mg

Beta-carotene: 700 µg

Lutein and zeaxanthin: 384 µg

Omega-3 fatty acids: 2 g

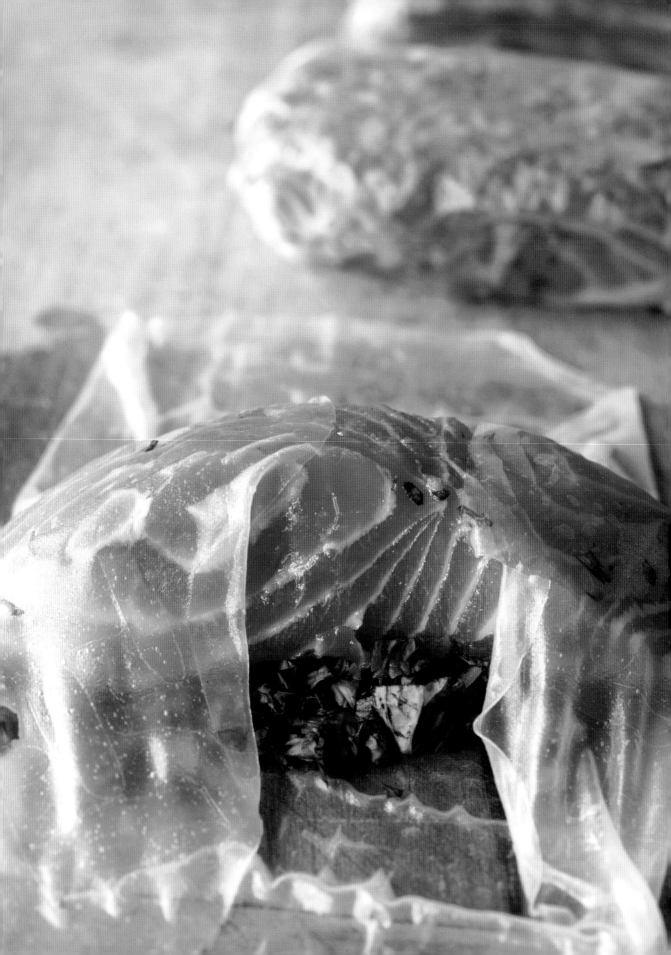

Pigs in a Blanket

SERVES 8

Pigs in a Blanket in some regions means a '50s-style appetizer with crescent rolls and hot dogs, but in Pittsburgh, Pennsylvania, it refers to stuffed cabbage (much healthier, thanks to cabbage's fiber and beta-carotene). This recipe from Dr. Johanna Seddon's mother is a traditional Polish recipe for golumpkies. You might make a big batch, since they freeze beautifully.

½   cup long-grain white rice (or brown rice or barley)

1   medium onion, chopped

1   medium cabbage (about 3 pounds)

1   pound lean ground pork or beef

1   large egg, beaten

One   15-ounce can tomato sauce, or for thicker sauce use tomato paste

Soak the rice in 2 cups of hot water for about 30 minutes to soften and remove some of the starch. Heat ¼ cup of water in a large skillet over medium heat. Add the onion and cook until soft, 3 to 5 minutes. Drain well.

Meanwhile, core the cabbage, place it in a large pot over high heat, and add water to cover. Boil for 15 minutes, or until pliable and soft. Drain and allow to cool completely. Carefully remove one leaf at a time. Using a sharp knife, remove the hard center vein from the leaves. Set the cabbage aside.

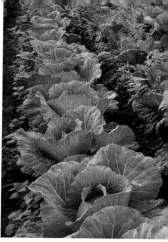

Drain the rice and add it to a large bowl with the meat, onion, and beaten egg. Gently mix them all together. Place a palm-sized amount into the center of a cabbage leaf and fold the leaf over, tucking in the sides to keep the meat mixture inside.

Place some extra cabbage leaves on the bottom of the pot and add the cabbage rolls packed tightly together. Add the tomato sauce and enough water to cover the cabbage rolls. Place additional cabbage leaves on top of the rolls. Simmer over medium heat for 50 to 60 minutes. (Keep an eye on them, making sure the bottoms of the leaves do not burn.)

Nutritional Profile

Serving size: 1 cabbage roll

Calories: 339

Protein: 41 g

Fiber: 6 g

Fat: 8 g

Saturated fat: 2 g

Sodium: 459 mg

Vitamin A: 264 IU

Vitamin C: 118 mg

Vitamin D: 12 IU

Vitamin E: 2 IU

Zinc: 4 mg

Beta-carotene: 138 µg

Lutein and zeaxanthin: 44 µg

Lycopene: 7,431 µg

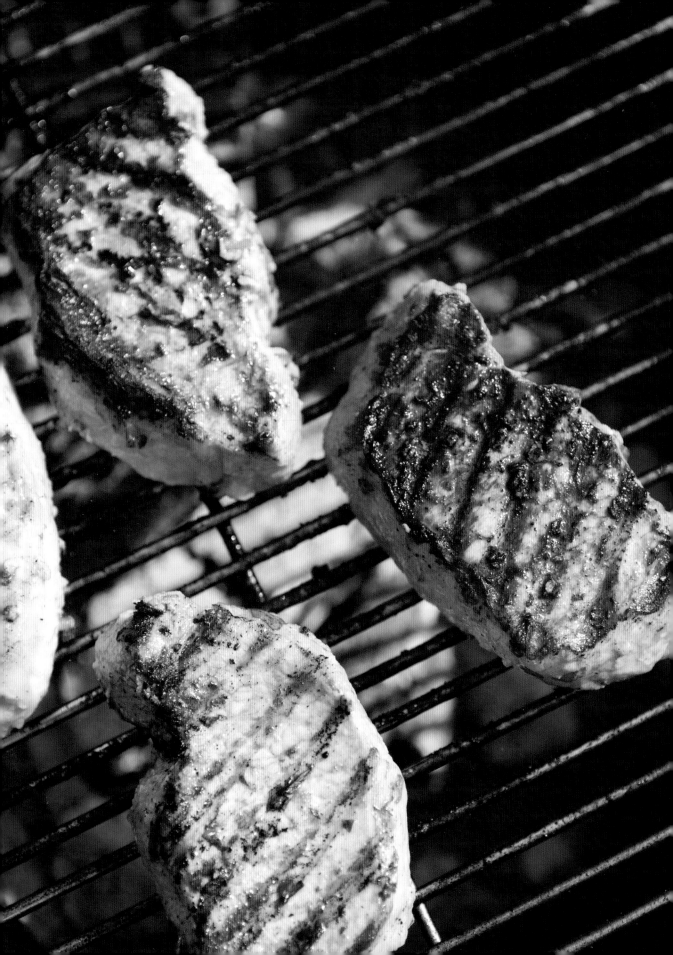

Garlic-Lime Pork Chops

SERVES 4

Pork provides thiamin, riboflavin, niacin, and phosphorus, not to mention protein. Serve with parsleyed brown rice.

Juice and zest of 2 limes
2 garlic cloves, minced
½ teaspoon hot pepper flakes
⅓ cup extra virgin olive oil
¼ teaspoon sea salt
¼ teaspoon freshly ground black pepper
2 tablespoons freshly chopped cilantro
2 tablespoons freshly chopped basil
1 teaspoon minced fresh ginger
4 lean ½-inch-thick boneless pork chops (about 1 to 1½ pounds)

Whisk together all ingredients except the pork chops in a bowl. Add the pork chops and marinate, covered, in the refrigerator for at least 3 hours or overnight.

When ready to serve, bring the pork chops to room temperature and prepare a grill. Cook over medium-high heat just until cooked through, about 6 minutes per side, or until a meat thermometer reads 145°F.

Nutritional Profile

Serving size: 1 pork chop

Calories: 602
Protein: 55 g
Fiber: 1 g
Fat: 40 g
Saturated fat: 8 g
Sodium: 348 mg
Vitamin A: 245 IU
Vitamin C: 6 mg
Vitamin D: 79 IU
Vitamin E: 4 IU
Zinc: 7 mg
Beta-carotene: 127 µg
Lutein and zeaxanthin: 105 µg

Stuffed Cabbage

SERVES 8

G rown in ancient Greece, cabbage was considered a
panacea for treating various conditions, for good
reason—cabbage helps eye health and heart health
and contributes to weight-loss efforts. This cousin to
golumpkies is richly flavored.

1	large savoy cabbage
1	pound lean (94 percent) ground turkey
1	pound Italian sweet turkey sausage
2	garlic cloves, minced
2	cups cooked barley
3	celery stalks, finely chopped
½	red bell pepper, cored, seeded, and chopped
½	green bell pepper, cored, seeded, and chopped
1	cup chopped yellow onion
2	teaspoons freshly chopped thyme
¼	cup freshly chopped parsley
2	tablespoons freshly snipped chives
1	tablespoon paprika
1	teaspoon sea salt
½	teaspoon freshly ground black pepper
	Olive oil, for the baking dish
One	28-ounce can diced tomatoes
2	cups homemade chicken stock or reduced-fat, low-sodium chicken broth

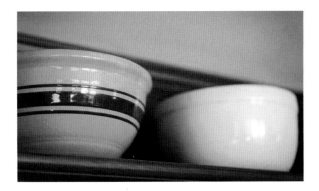

In a large pot, bring several cups of water to a boil. Remove the cabbage core, place the cabbage into the boiling water, and cook for 10 minutes on medium-high heat. Remove the cabbage from the pot and drain. When cool, separate the leaves and cut out the hard vein, taking care to preserve the shape of the leaves.

In a large bowl, combine the turkey, turkey sausage, garlic, barley, celery, red and green bell peppers, onion, thyme, parsley, chives, paprika, salt, and black pepper, stirring to mix well.

Preheat the oven to 375°F. Coat a 9 by 13-inch roasting pan with olive oil.

With a cabbage leaf in your hand, spoon ⅓ cup of the turkey mixture into the leaf and roll it, tucking in the sides. Place it seam side down in the pan. Repeat with the remaining leaves, filling the pan with a single layer of rolls.

In a small bowl, combine the tomatoes and chicken stock and pour over the cabbage. Season to taste, cover, and bake for 2 hours, or until the cabbage is tender.

Nutritional Profile

Serving size: 2 cabbage rolls

Calories: 419
Protein: 29 g
Fiber: 12 g
Fat: 13 g
Saturated fat: 2 g
Sodium: 1,070 mg
Vitamin A: 1,833 IU
Vitamin C: 55 mg
Vitamin E: 2 IU
Zinc: 2 mg
Beta-carotene: 953 µg
Lutein and zeaxanthin: 479 µg

Mini Meatloaves

SERVES 8

These individual meatloaves satisfy any meat lover, but they are filled with a surprising amount of healthy vegetables. For easy prep, use a food processor to make your bread crumbs, then chop the carrots, celery, onion, garlic, and spinach, taking care not to overprocess. They should still retain their shape and not give off too much water.

TOPPING

- ¼ cup ketchup
- 1 tablespoon light brown sugar
- ½ teaspoon powdered mustard

MEATLOAF

- 1 cup freshly made white bread crumbs
- 1 cup finely diced carrots
- ½ cup finely diced celery
- ½ cup finely diced onion
- 2 garlic cloves, minced
- One 9-ounce package frozen chopped spinach, thawed and drained well
- 2 large eggs
- ½ cup ketchup
- 2 teaspoons powdered mustard
- 1 teaspoon Italian seasoning
- 1 teaspoon sea salt
- 1 teaspoon freshly ground black pepper
- 1½ pounds combination of ground turkey breast, lean ground beef, and/or pork

Preheat the oven to 350°F. Line a rimmed baking sheet with aluminum foil. To prepare the topping, combine the ketchup, brown sugar and mustard in a bowl. Set aside.

To prepare the meatloaf, combine the bread crumbs, carrots, celery, onion, garlic, and spinach in a large bowl. In a separate bowl, beat the eggs. Add the ketchup, mustard, Italian seasoning, salt, and pepper and stir well to combine. Gently stir in the meat. Then gently stir in the bread crumb mixture.

Form into 8 equal-sized small loaves and place on the prepared baking sheet. Brush with the topping. Bake for 25 to 30 minutes, until a meat thermometer registers 160°F. Remove to cool just slightly, about 5 minutes, before serving.

Nutritional Profile

Serving size: 1 meatloaf

Calories: 232
Protein: 23 g
Fiber: 2 g
Fat: 6 g
Saturated fat: 2 g
Sodium: 850 mg
Vitamin A: 3,922 IU
Vitamin C: 5 mg
Vitamin D: 14 IU
Vitamin E: 1 IU
Zinc: 2 mg
Beta-carotene: 1,458 µg
Lutein and zeaxanthin: 125 µg
Lycopene: 2,566 µg

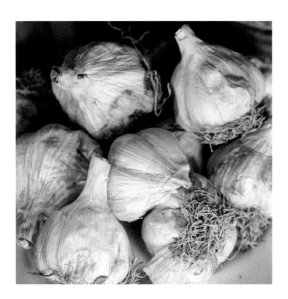

Pumpkin Pappardelle

SERVES 4

The drizzle of pomegranate, high in beta-carotene, adds a bold accent, as well as an unexpected contrast of flavor to this recipe from Canyon Ranch. Pomegranate juice concentrate is available at health food stores and in gourmet markets.

- 2 tablespoons extra virgin olive oil
- 1 small shallot, minced
- 3 garlic cloves, minced
- 1 small butternut or calabaza squash, peeled, seeded, and diced (about ½ cup)
- 1 cup vegetable stock
- ¾ cup canned pumpkin (not pumpkin pie filling)
  - Pinch of ground cinnamon
  - Pinch of sea salt
  - Pinch of freshly ground black pepper
- 6 ounces fresh fettuccine
- 4 teaspoons chopped macadamia nuts
- 2 tablespoons pomegranate juice concentrate

In a large sauté pan, heat the olive oil over medium heat and sauté the shallot and garlic until the shallot is translucent, 3 to 5 minutes. Add the butternut squash and sauté until tender, 15 to 20 minutes.

Deglaze the pan (moistening and scraping up the brown bits) with the vegetable stock. Add the pumpkin (undrained), cinnamon, salt, and pepper and cook until heated through.

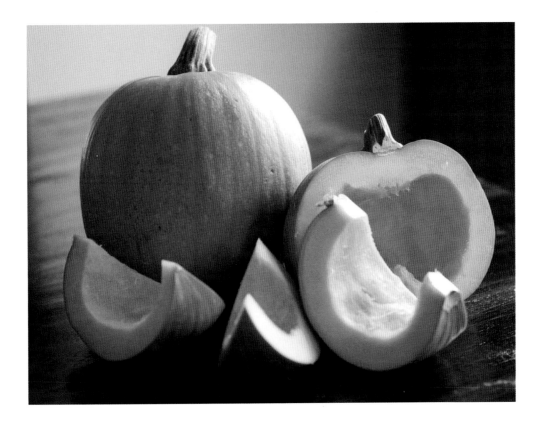

Cook the pasta according to package directions and stir it into the pumpkin mixture.

Evenly divide the pumpkin and pasta mixture among four large bowls.
Top each serving with 1 teaspoon of chopped macadamia nuts. Drizzle ½ tablespoon of pomegranate juice concentrate over each serving.

Nutritional Profile

Serving Size: 2½ cups

Calories: 265
Protein: 7 g
Fiber: 3 g
Fat: 11 g
Saturated fat: 2 g
Sodium: 370 mg
Vitamin A: 9,184 IU
Vitamin C: 7 mg
Vitamin D: 23 IU
Vitamin E: 2 IU
Beta-carotene: 3,928 µg
Lutein and zeaxanthin: 2 µg

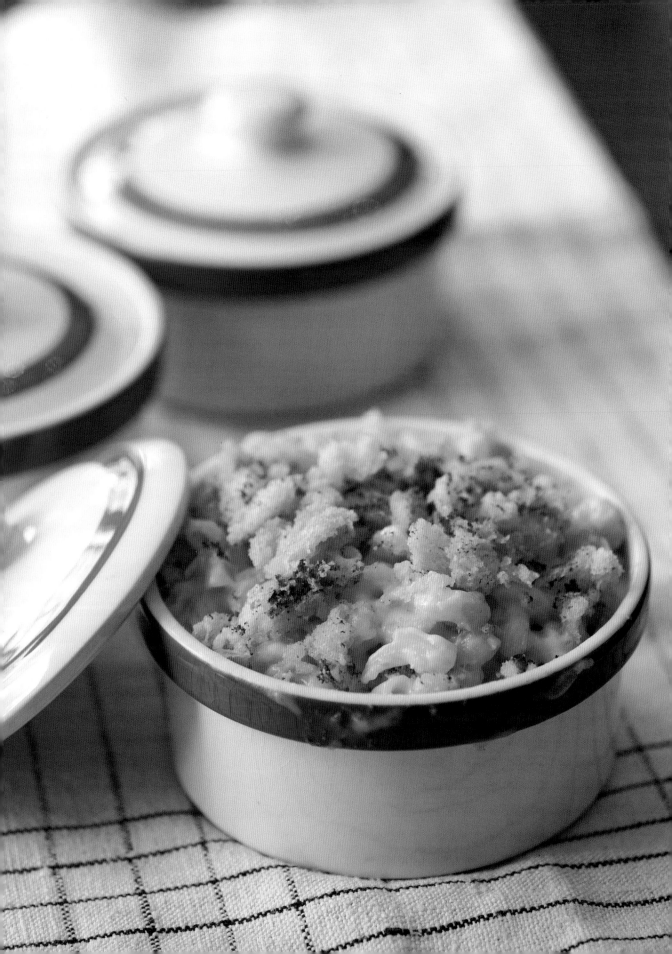

Macaroni and Cheese

L ike other orange vegetables, carrots are high in beta-carotene, which when absorbed by the body converts to vitamin A—important to eye health. Here, shredded carrots complement this classic dish but don't overwhelm it; you could also substitute other vegetables such as broccoli, spinach, or zucchini (just blanch with the pasta).

8	ounces elbow macaroni
2½	cups coarsely grated carrots
¼	cup (½ stick) unsalted butter, divided
3	tablespoons all-purpose flour
1¾	cups milk, heated
3	cups grated sharp cheddar cheese
1	teaspoon sea salt
½	teaspoon powdered mustard
½	teaspoon freshly ground black pepper
1	cup fresh bread crumbs
½	cup freshly grated Parmesan cheese

Preheat the oven to 400°F. Lightly coat an 8 by 8-inch baking pan with nonstick cooking spray.

Cook the macaroni according to the package directions until al dente (just firm). Add the carrots 3 to 4 minutes before the pasta is finished. Using a slotted spoon, skim off any foam that rises to the surface. Drain and set aside.

CONTINUED

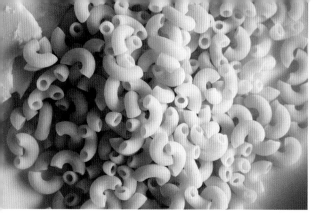

Meanwhile, in a saucepan over medium heat, melt 3 tablespoons of butter. Whisk in the flour until it's completely incorporated, about 1 minute, whisking constantly. Add the milk and cook until thickened, whisking constantly. Reduce the heat and cook for 3 to 5 minutes, whisking often.

Remove from the heat and add the cheddar cheese, salt, mustard, and pepper. Stir until the cheese has melted. Add the pasta mixture and stir well to combine. Transfer to the baking pan.

Melt the remaining tablespoon of butter. In a small bowl, mix the bread crumbs with the melted butter. Stir in the Parmesan. Sprinkle on top of the macaroni mixture. Bake for 15 to 20 minutes, until the top is golden brown. Remove from the oven and let cool just slightly before serving.

Nutritional Profile

Serving size: 2 cups

Calories: 610

Protein: 27 g

Fiber: 3 g

Fat: 32 g

Saturated fat: 18 g

Sodium: 1,217 mg

Vitamin A: 9,503 IU

Vitamin C: 3 mg

Vitamin D: 21 IU

Vitamin E: 1 IU

Zinc: 1 mg

Beta-carotene: 4,237 µg

Lutein and zeaxanthin: 132 µg

Red Curry Vegetables with Coconut Sauce

SERVES 4

Canyon Ranch knows how to dress up a plate of vegetables. The edamame is a smart addition; a star legume, this soybean offers complete protein, with all the amino acid building blocks, as well as antioxidants. Grapes add a sweet touch, and recent studies have suggested they may help stave off age-related macular degeneration.

1 medium zucchini, diced (about 1 cup)

1 medium yellow squash, diced (about 1 cup)

½ yellow or red bell pepper, diced (about ½ cup)

1 cup diced fresh pineapple

¾ cup seedless red grapes, halved

1 cup shelled edamame

COCONUT SAUCE

One 14-ounce can light coconut milk

1 cup water

2 tablespoons low-sodium tamari sauce

2 tablespoons turbinado sugar

3 tablespoons freshly squeezed lime juice

¼ cup prepared Thai red curry paste

4 Kaffir lime leaves

1⅓ cups cooked brown rice

½ cup toasted pistachios, chopped

CONTINUED

In a large bowl, toss together the zucchini, squash, bell peppers, pineapple, grapes, and edamame. In a medium bowl, mix together all the ingredients for the Coconut Sauce. Set it aside.

In a large sauté pan, sauté the red curry paste over low heat until slightly caramelized. Add the vegetable mixture and sauté until the vegetables are slightly cooked. Increase the heat to high and add the Coconut Sauce and lime leaves. Bring to a boil, reduce to a simmer, and continue simmering until reduced by half.

Place ⅓ cup of brown rice in the bottom of each of four bowls. Evenly divide the vegetables and sauce among the bowls. Top each serving with 2 tablespoons of toasted pistachios.

Nutritional Profile

Serving size: 2 cups

Calories: 491
Protein: 14 g
Fiber: 8 g
Fat: 15 g
Saturated fat: 4 g
Sodium: 418 mg
Vitamin A: 929 IU
Vitamin C: 69 mg
Vitamin E: 2 IU
Zinc: 2 mg
Beta-carotene: 487 µg
Lutein and zeaxanthin: 2,328 µg

"The act of putting into your mouth what the earth has grown is perhaps your most direct interaction with the earth."
— *Frances Moore Lappé*

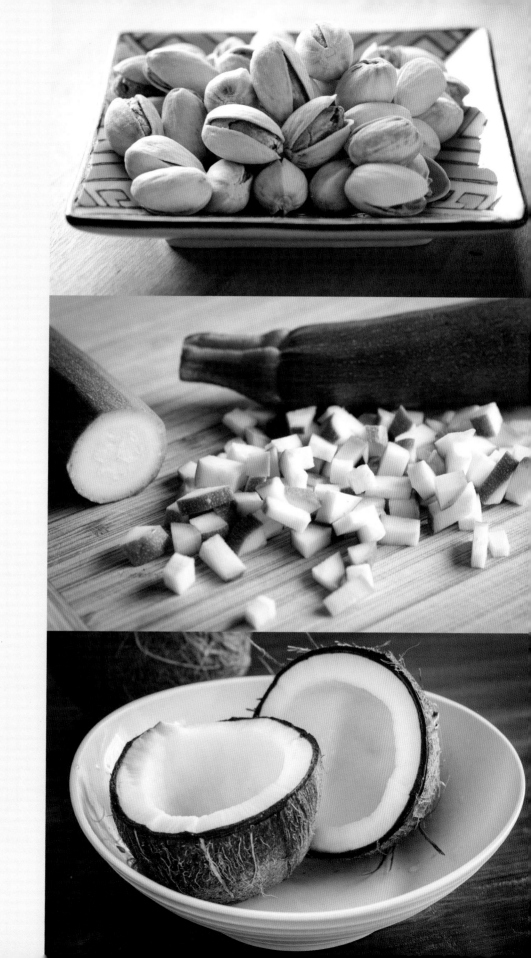

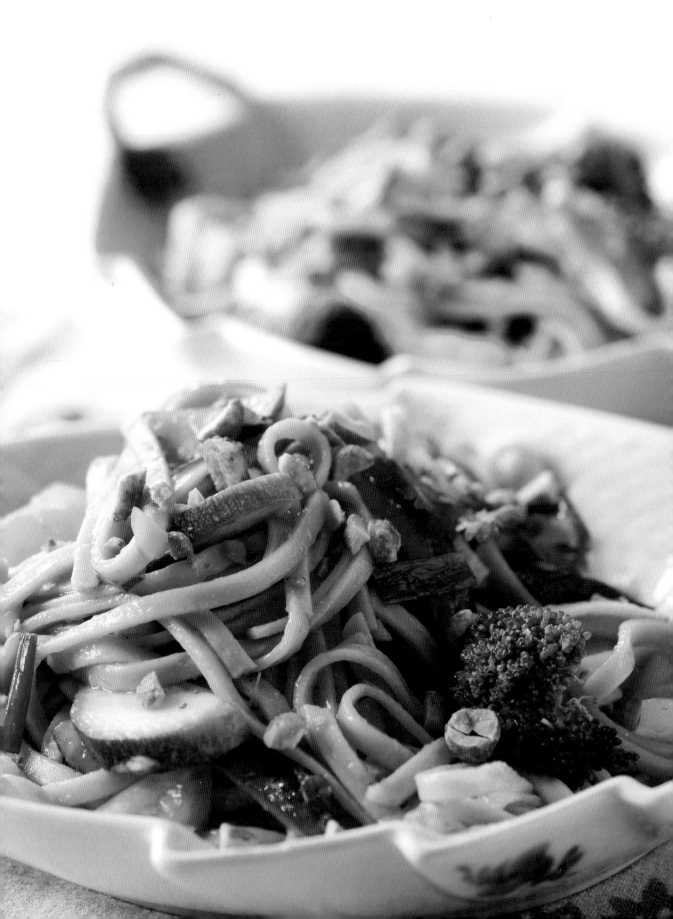

Spicy Udon Noodles

SERVES 4

A hit with guests at the Lake Austin Spa Resort in Texas, this dish has just enough heat to get your attention. This mosaic of multicolored vegetables—good for cancer prevention, heart health, and eye health—is doused in a pungent sauce before being tossed with fresh herbs.

	Zest and juice of 1 orange
2	tablespoons hoisin sauce
1	tablespoon low-sodium soy sauce
1	tablespoon Asian chili paste
1½	tablespoons sugar
1½	tablespoons rice wine vinegar
1	tablespoon toasted sesame oil
1	tablespoon canola oil
1½	tablespoons minced garlic
1½	tablespoons minced fresh ginger
6	cups mixed cut raw stir-fry vegetables (broccoli, bok choy, zucchini, onion, scallion, red bell peppers, carrots)
3	cups cooked udon noodles (9 ounces dry)
¼	cup freshly chopped basil leaves
¼	cup freshly chopped mint leaves
¼	cup freshly chopped cilantro leaves
2	tablespoons chopped dry-roasted peanuts, for garnish

CONTINUED

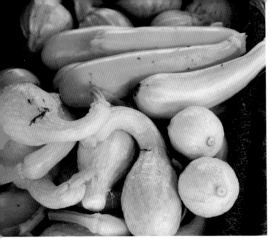

Combine the orange zest and juice, hoisin sauce, soy sauce, chili paste, sugar, and vinegar in a bowl; set it aside. Combine the sesame oil and canola oil in a small bowl.

Heat 2 teaspoons of the oil mixture in a skillet over high heat. Add the garlic and ginger and stir-fry until they begin to color, about 2 minutes. Add the mixed vegetables and stir-fry until crisp-tender, 1 to 2 minutes. Add the noodles and reserved sauce. Cook for 1 minute. Add the basil, mint, and cilantro; toss to mix. Serve hot; garnish with the peanuts.

Nutritional Profile

Serving size: 3 cups

Calories: 453
Protein: 14 g
Fiber: 7 g
Fat: 11 g
Saturated fat: 1 g
Sodium: 608 mg
Vitamin A: 1,245 IU
Vitamin C: 41 mg
Vitamin E: 1 IU
Zinc: 1 mg
Beta-carotene: 93 µg
Lutein and zeaxanthin: 170 µg

Jacques Pépin's Provence Pizza

SERVES 6

Even pizza can be made in a way that's good for your eyes! Depending on your oven, you may have to bake longer than indicated to crisp the bottom. If you use a pizza stone, the pizzas will get crustier on the bottom. For added crispness, make the dough as thin as possible.

CRUST

- ⅔ cup warm water (110–115°F)
- 1 package active dry yeast (about 2 teaspoons)
- ¼ teaspoon sugar
- 2 cups all-purpose flour
- ¼ teaspoon sea salt

TOPPINGS

- 4 large onions, peeled and thinly sliced (about 6 cups)
- 1 cup water
- 1 tablespoon extra virgin olive oil
- 1 teaspoon salt
- 1 teaspoon freshly ground black pepper
- 4 garlic cloves, peeled, crushed, and finely chopped (2 teaspoons)
- 2 ripe medium tomatoes, seeded and coarsely chopped
- 1 small zucchini, washed, trimmed, and cut crosswise into ¼-inch slices (1 cup)
- 8 ounces button mushrooms, washed and cut into ¼-inch slices
- 1 medium red bell pepper (4 ounces), cored, seeded, and cut crosswise into thin rings (about ¾ cup)
- 1 medium green bell pepper (4 ounces), cored, seeded, and cut crosswise into thin rings (about ¾ cup)
- 4 ounces part-skim mozzarella cheese, shredded

CONTINUED

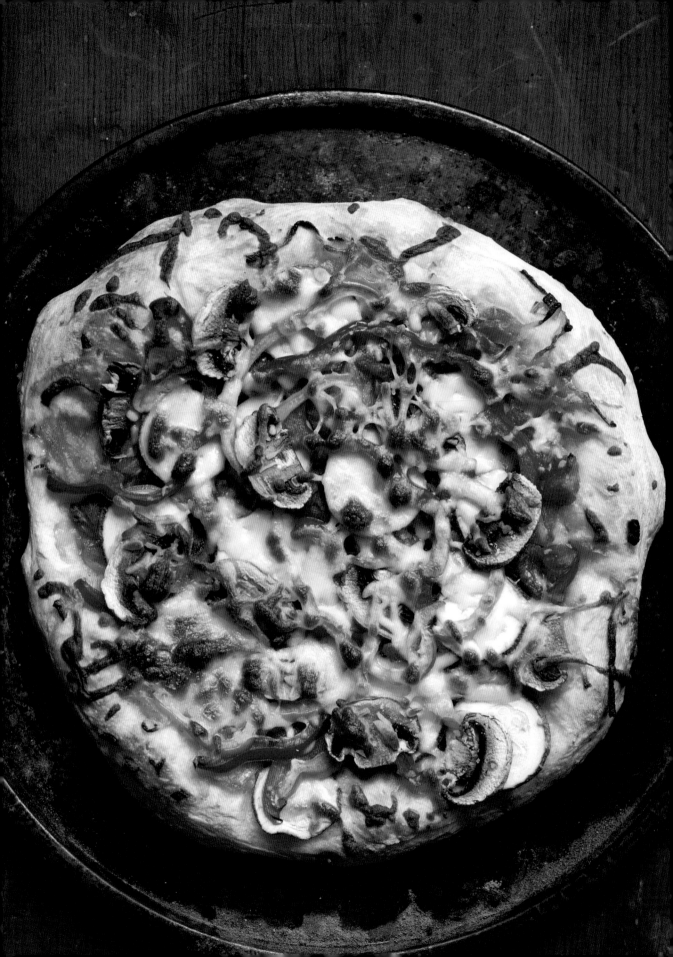

TO MAKE THE CRUST: Place the water, yeast, and sugar in a mixing bowl. Stir well and let rest for 5 minutes. Add the flour and salt; mix with the dough hook of an electric mixer at low speed for 3 minutes.

Place the dough in a large bowl, cover the bowl with plastic wrap, and set it aside in a warm place (75 to 80°F) for about 2 hours or until the dough has doubled in volume. (When the dough is ready, touching it firmly will leave an indentation.)

While the dough is rising, spray 2 cookie sheets or pizza pans lightly with nonstick cooking spray and set them aside.

TO MAKE THE TOPPINGS: Place the onions, water, oil, salt, and pepper in a large skillet or saucepan. Bring the mixture to a boil over high heat, cover, and reduce the heat to medium. Boil for about 12 minutes, until most of the water has evaporated. Uncover and continue to cook, stirring often, until the onions begin to brown. Add the garlic, mix well, and set the pan aside off the heat.

After the dough has doubled in volume, punch it down gently and divide it in half. Place half the dough on one of the prepared sheets or pans and shape it into a 10-inch round, with the edges slightly thicker than the center. (The dough will have a tendency to spring back; you will need to push and press on it firmly to extend it.) Repeat this procedure with the remaining dough, spreading it out on the other prepared sheet or pan.

Arrange the tomatoes evenly over the dough and layer on the zucchini, mushrooms, red bell pepper, and green pepper. Divide the onion mixture between the pizzas and top with the mozzarella.

Preheat the oven to 425°F.

Bake the pizzas for 25 to 30 minutes, until the crust on each is brown throughout. Let the pizzas cool for 3 to 4 minutes, cut them into wedges, and serve.

Nutritional Profile

Serving size: 2 small slices

Calories: 290

Protein: 12 g

Fiber: 4 g

Fat: 7 g

Saturated fat: 3 g

Sodium: 1,253 mg

Vitamin A: 900 IU

Vitamin C: 44 mg

Vitamin D: 3 IU

Vitamin E: 1 IU

Zinc: 1 mg

Beta-carotene: 367 µg

Lutein and zeaxanthin: 444 µg

Lycopene: 79 µg

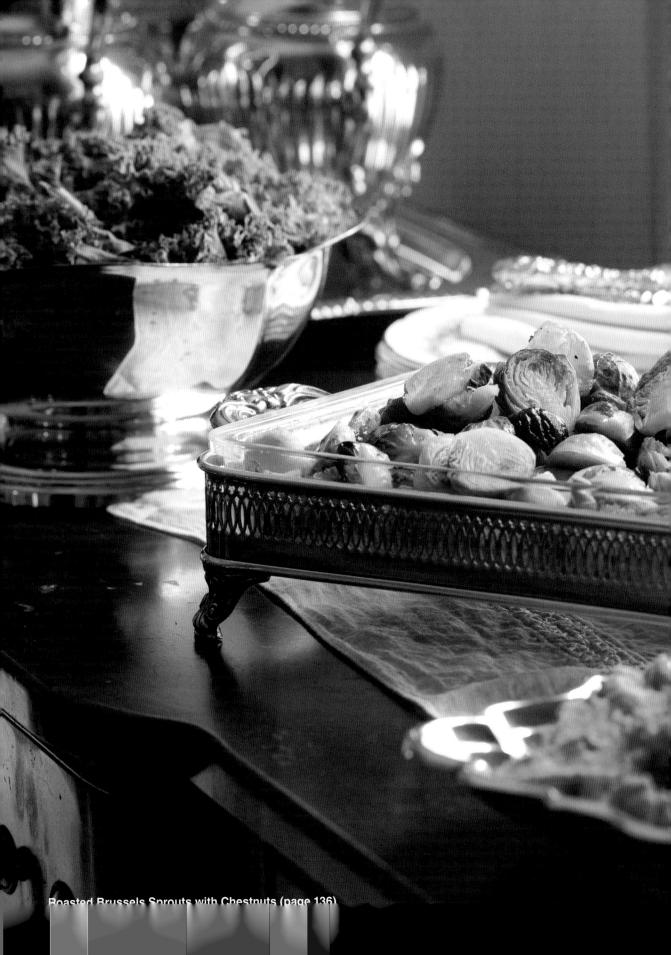

Roasted Brussels Sprouts with Chestnuts (page 136)

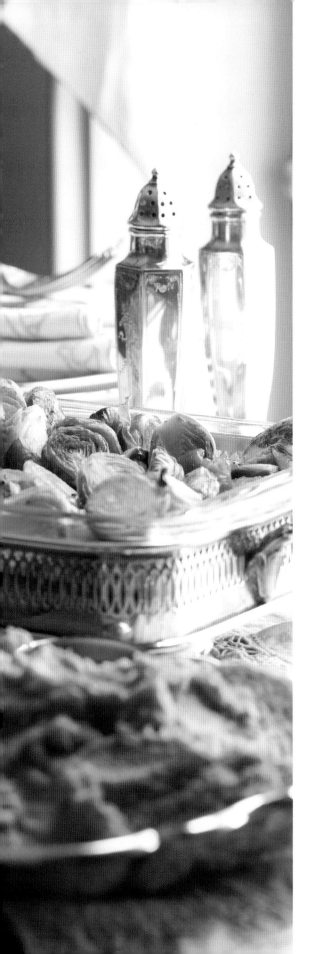

Side Dishes

Roasted Brussels Sprouts
   with Chestnuts

Sautéed Spinach
   with Shiitake Mushrooms

Alice Waters's Cannellini Beans
   and Wilted Greens

Ina Garten's Confetti Corn

Roasted Tomatoes

Chez Panisse's Spicy Broccoli
   Vegetable Sauté

Broccoli with Sun-Dried
   Tomatoes and Pine Nuts

Okra and Tomatoes

Roasted Brussels Sprouts with Chestnuts

Named for the capital of Belgium, these tiny cabbages may have been developed in northern Europe as early as the sixth century, although their origin is debated by culinary scholars. They were brought to the States by French settlers in Louisiana, and Thomas Jefferson cultivated them at Monticello. Brussels sprouts are exceptionally rich in fiber, vitamins, minerals, and antioxidants.

2   pounds brussels sprouts, trimmed (about 4 cups)

¾   cup bottled halved chestnuts (not sweetened)

2   tablespoons olive oil

½   teaspoon kosher salt

¼   teaspoon coarsely ground black pepper

Pinch of cayenne

Preheat oven to 400°F. In a bowl, toss the sprouts and chestnuts with the olive oil, salt, black pepper, and cayenne. Spread in a single layer on a rimmed baking sheet with sides.

Bake until the sprouts are tender, 20 to 25 minutes, stirring after 10 minutes. Season to taste. Serve immediately.

Nutritional Profile

Serving size: 1 cup

Calories: 226

Protein: 6 g

Fiber: 10 g

Fat: 9 g

Saturated fat: 1 g

Sodium: 309 mg

Vitamin A: 1,135 IU

Vitamin C: 206 mg

Vitamin E: 2 IU

Beta-carotene: 669 µg

Lutein and zeaxanthin: 190 µg

Sautéed Spinach with Shiitake Mushrooms

SERVES 4

Important to the Chinese for thousands of years, shiitakes are tastier than button mushrooms and have an impressive nutritional profile. The fourteenth-century Chinese physician Wu-Rui described the shiitake as a food that accelerated "spirit" energy and warded off hunger. Just look at all the nutrients in this dish: lutein and zeaxanthin, not to mention the vitamins A, C, D, and E.

2 pounds fresh spinach, stemmed and coarsely chopped

2 tablespoons extra virgin olive oil

½ pound shiitake mushrooms, cleaned, stems removed, and sliced (3 cups)

3 garlic cloves, minced

½ teaspoon freshly chopped thyme

½ teaspoon sea salt

Freshly ground black pepper

¼ teaspoon freshly grated nutmeg

Nutritional Profile		
Serving size: 1 cup		
Calories: 139		
Protein: 8 g		
Fiber: 7 g		
Fat: 8 g		
Saturated fat: 1 g		
Sodium: 535 mg		
Vitamin A: 21,273 IU		
Vitamin C: 65 mg		
Vitamin D: 10 IU		
Vitamin E: 8 IU		
Zinc: 2 mg		
Beta-carotene: 12,763 µg		
Lutein and zeaxanthin: 27,666 µg		

Rinse the spinach and leave it in the colander.

Heat the olive oil in a skillet over medium-high heat and add shiitakes. Cook, stirring frequently, until they are seared and beginning to sweat, about 5 minutes.

Lower the heat to medium and add the garlic, thyme, salt, pepper, and nutmeg, continuing to stir until the mushrooms are tender, about 1 minute. Add damp spinach and stir until it's wilted, about 5 minutes. Remove from the heat and season to taste.

Alice Waters's Cannellini Beans and Wilted Greens

SERVES 6–8

This is an excellent side dish for roasted or grilled poultry and it is also a fine sauce for a sturdy pasta, such as penne. When the beans are tender, mash about half of them to thicken the sauce and then stir in the cooked pasta. Add a little more bean liquid if the mixture is too thick.

2	cups dried cannellini beans
	Bouquet garni (leafy celery stalk, thyme sprig, parsley sprig, and bay leaf tied together with twine or string)
1	onion, peeled
1	carrot, peeled
6	cups water or chicken stock
	Fine sea salt
1	large bunch chard, kale, spinach, mustard greens, or turnip greens (about 1 pound)
5 to 6	tablespoons olive oil
6	garlic cloves, minced
1	tablespoon freshly chopped rosemary leaves
	Freshly ground black pepper
	Extra virgin olive oil, for serving

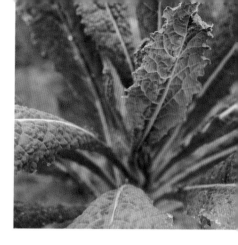

Soak the beans overnight. The next day, drain them and put them into a heavy-bottomed pot with the bouquet garni. Add the onion and carrot. Cover with water or stock and bring to a boil. Reduce to a simmer, skimming off any foam that forms on the surface. Cook the beans until very tender, from 45 minutes to 2 hours, depending on the age of the beans and how long they were soaked. Salt the beans generously once they start to soften. When they're fully cooked, remove them from the heat.

While the beans are cooking, wash, trim, and chop the greens. Drain the beans, reserving the liquid. Gently sauté the garlic in the 5 to 6 tablespoons olive oil with the rosemary until fragrant, about 1 minute. Add the beans and about 1 cup of their cooking liquid; simmer about 5 minutes, until some of the beans have crumbled apart.

Add the greens to the beans, and stew together, uncovered, until the greens are wilted and tender. Add more of the bean liquid, if needed, to keep the vegetables moist and a little soupy. Taste and adjust the seasoning with salt and pepper. Serve with olive oil drizzled over the surface.

Nutritional Profile

Serving size: 1½ cups

Calories: 110

Protein: 8 g

Fiber: 6 g

Fat: 10 g

Saturated fat: 1 g

Sodium: 340 mg

Vitamin A: 7,804 IU

Vitamin C: 21 mg

Vitamin E: 4 IU

Beta-carotene: 4,498 µg

Lutein and zeaxanthin: 7,932 µg

Ina Garten's Confetti Corn

SERVES 6

In late summer, when corn is bountiful, Ina Garten tosses kernels with other vegetables and herbs that are available on Eastern Long Island, creating a casual fresh dish that's a colorful accompaniment to a grilling menu. In this recipe, she suggests cooking the corn as soon as possible after it's picked because sugar turns to starch quickly.

2   tablespoons good olive oil

½   cup chopped red onion

1   small orange bell pepper, ½-inch diced

2   tablespoons unsalted butter

    Kernels cut from 5 ears yellow or white corn (4 cups)

1½ teaspoons kosher salt

1   teaspoon freshly ground black pepper

2   tablespoons julienned fresh basil, minced fresh chives, and/or minced fresh parsley

Heat the olive oil over medium heat in a large sauté pan. Add the onion and sauté for 5 minutes, until the onion is soft. Stir in the bell pepper and sauté for 2 more minutes.

Add the butter to the pan and allow it to melt. Over medium heat, add the corn, salt, and pepper and cook, stirring occasionally, for 5 to 7 minutes, until the corn just loses its starchiness. Season to taste, gently stir in the basil or other green herbs, and serve hot.

Nutritional Profile

Serving size: 1 cup

Calories: 175

Protein: 4 g

Fiber: 3 g

Fat: 10 g

Saturated fat: 3 g

Sodium: 497 mg

Vitamin A: 199 IU

Vitamin C: 37 mg

Vitamin D: 3 IU

Vitamin E: 1 IU

Zinc: 1 mg

Beta-carotene: 56 µg

Lutein and zeaxanthin: 87 µg

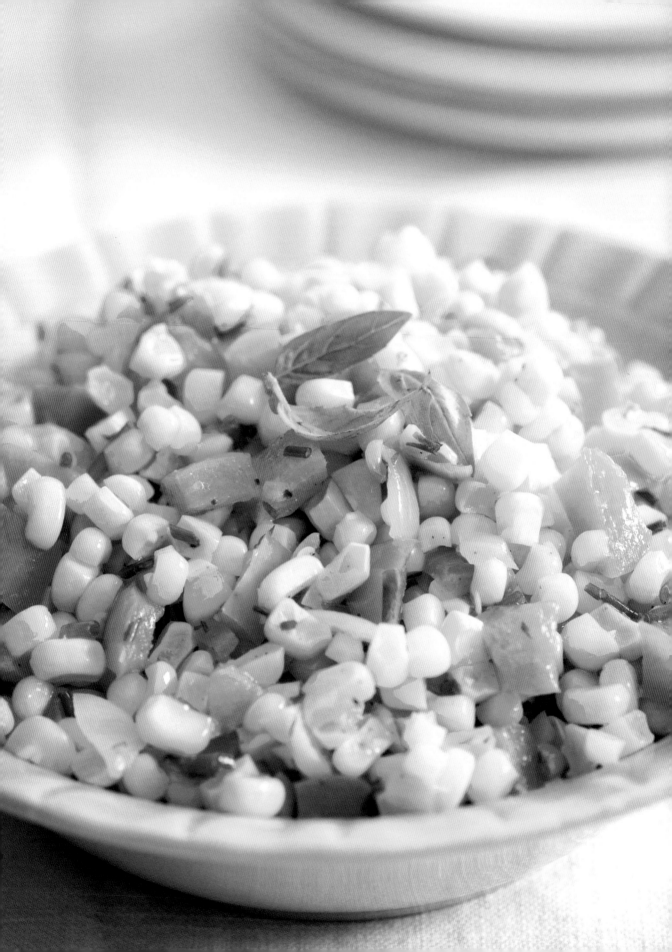

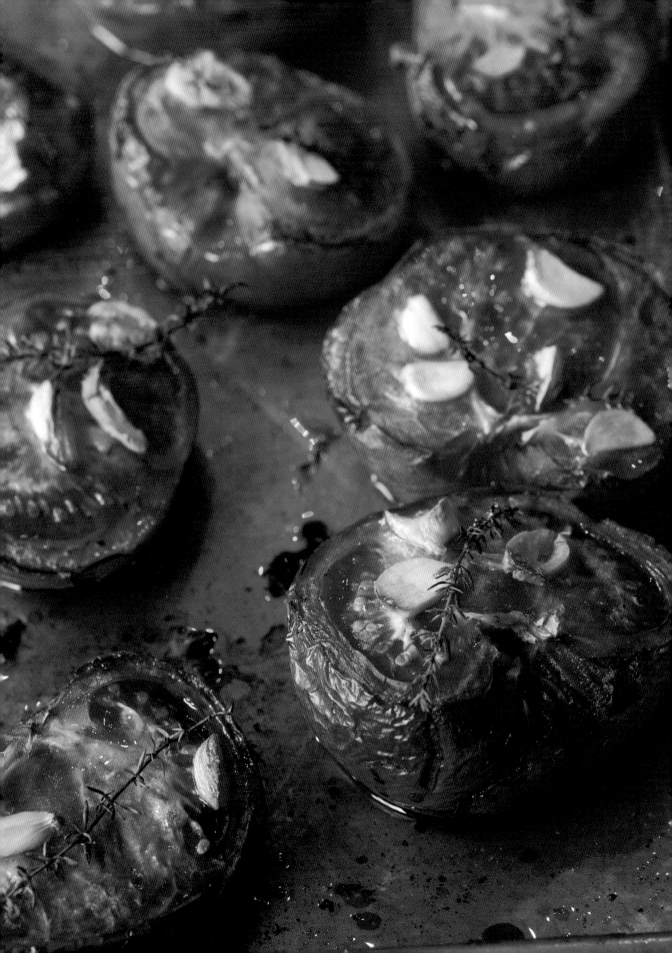

Roasted Tomatoes

SERVES 4

A lively accompaniment to chicken or pork, roasted tomatoes are eminently versatile—served with eggs on grilled bread, coarsely chopped on pasta or pizza, or in a toasted sandwich. Research indicates that tomatoes are one of the top foods for eye health, so enjoy them year-round by preserving them during the summer months. Cooked, they freeze well. Or make a big batch, place the container in the refrigerator, and eat them all week.

4   large tomatoes, halved
    Olive oil
2   garlic cloves, thinly sliced
    Fine sea salt
    Freshly ground black pepper

Preheat the oven to 325°F. Place tomatoes, cut side up, on a rimmed baking sheet or shallow baking dish. Brush with olive oil and top with slivers of garlic. Sprinkle with salt and pepper. Bake for 1 hour and 15 minutes, or until roasted and the garlic is golden. Serve immediately.

Nutritional Profile

Serving size: 2 tomato halves

Calories: 66
Protein: 2 g
Fiber: 2 g
Fat: 4 g
Saturated fat: 1 g
Sodium: 710 mg
Vitamin A: 1,519 IU
Vitamin C: 25 mg
Vitamin E: 2 IU
Beta-carotene: 819 µg
Lutein and zeaxanthin: 227 µg
Lycopene: 4,683 µg

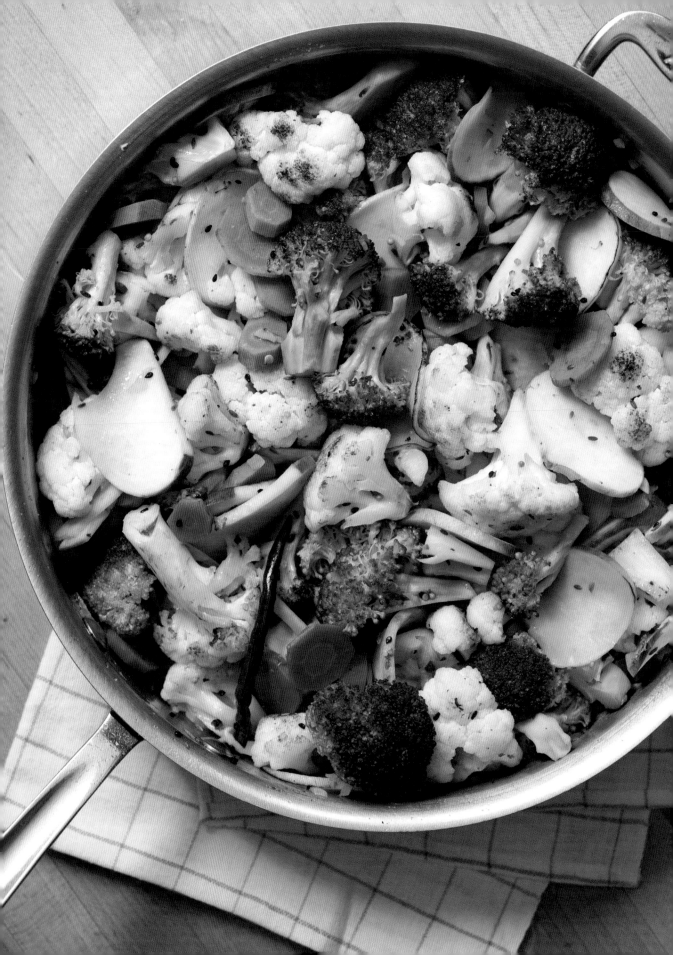

Chez Panisse's Spicy Broccoli Vegetable Sauté

SERVES 4

From the famed Berkeley, California, restaurant, this India-inspired dish goes well with saffron rice and cucumber raita. While the combination of vegetables may vary, broccoli is often a main ingredient and a good source of carotenoids.

2 carrots, peeled and sliced

3 tablespoons clarified butter or peanut oil

1 pound cauliflower, cut into florets

2 small dried chile peppers

4 curry leaves (optional)

½ pound baby turnips, sliced

1 medium head broccoli, cut into florets

1 small onion, finely diced

   Sea salt

   Freshly ground black pepper

½ teaspoon cumin seeds

1½ teaspoons mustard seeds

1 teaspoon black onion seeds

1 small knob fresh ginger, cut into julienne (about 2 teaspoons)

1 serrano pepper, finely chopped

4 garlic cloves, minced

   A few cilantro sprigs for garnish

CONTINUED

Parboil the carrots for about a minute, then drain. Heat the clarified butter in a large sauté pan. When it is hot, add the cauliflower and sauté until it has browned slightly. Add the dried chile peppers and the curry leaves, if you have them. Continue to sauté over medium heat, adding in succession the turnip slices, broccoli florets, and onion, tossing regularly so everything cooks evenly.

Salt and pepper the vegetables and add the cumin seeds, mustard seeds, and black onion seeds. Keep tossing, letting the seeds pop: this removes their bitterness and releases more flavor. Add the carrots, julienned ginger, chopped serrano pepper, and garlic. Taste and adjust the seasoning; the dish should be spicy. Garnish with cilantro sprigs and serve.

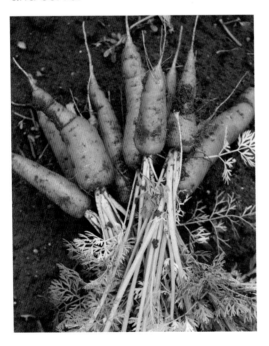

Nutritional Profile

Serving size: 1 cup

Calories: 189

Protein: 5 g

Fiber: 7 g

Fat: 12 g

Saturated fat: 2 g

Sodium: 293 mg

Vitamin A: 6,804 IU

Vitamin C: 109 mg

Vitamin E: 2 IU

Zinc: 1 mg

Beta-carotene: 3,450 µg

Lutein and zeaxanthin: 650 µg

Broccoli with Sun-Dried Tomatoes and Pine Nuts

SERVES 6

With broccoli, as with most vegetables, the deeper the color, the denser the nutrition. Broccoli is a good source of vitamin C, lutein, and zeaxanthin.

1 large head broccoli, cut into florets (4 cups)

¼ cup extra virgin olive oil, divided

2 tablespoons balsamic vinegar

1 garlic clove, minced

½ teaspoon sea salt

Freshly ground black pepper

2 sun-dried tomatoes in oil, drained and slivered

2 tablespoons pine nuts, toasted

Preheat the oven to 350°F. In a bowl, toss the broccoli with 1 tablespoon of olive oil and spread it in a single layer on a rimmed baking sheet. Bake until the florets are tender and crisp, about 20 minutes.

Meanwhile, in a small bowl, whisk together the vinegar, garlic, remaining 3 tablespoons of olive oil, salt, and pepper. Toss the broccoli with the dressing and sun-dried tomatoes, then with the pine nuts. Serve hot or at room temperature. Season to taste.

Nutritional Profile

Serving size: ¾ cup

Calories: 124

Protein: 2 g

Fiber: 2 g

Fat: 12 g

Saturated fat: 1 g

Sodium: 250 mg

Vitamin A: 1,435 IU

Vitamin C: 45 mg

Vitamin E: 2 IU

Beta-carotene: 1 µg

Lutein and zeaxanthin: 1 µg

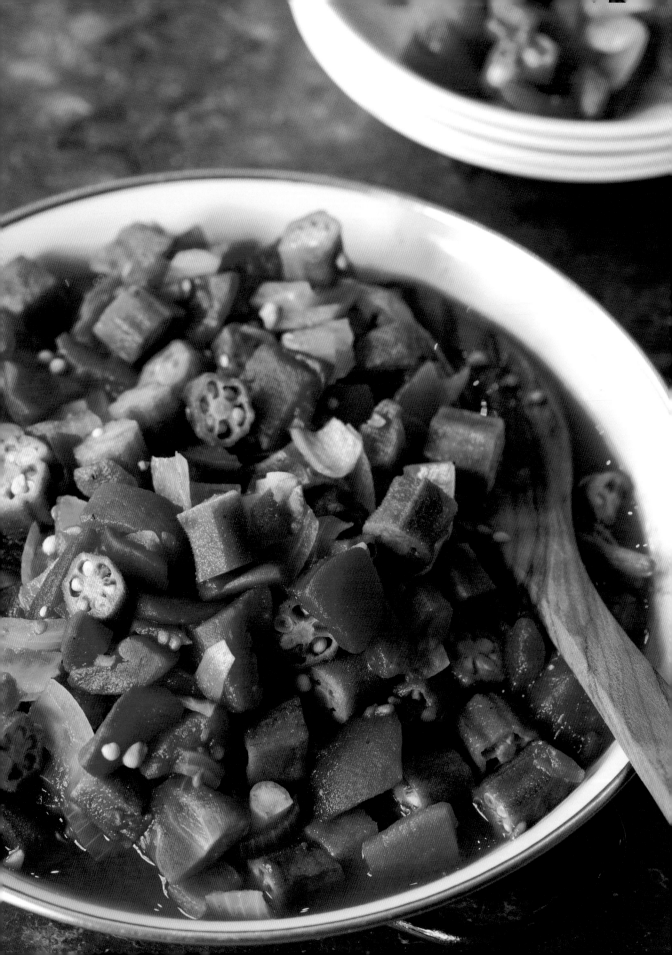

Okra and Tomatoes

SERVES 4–6

Jennifer's Oklahoma mother-in-law taught her about cooking okra, and she's come to love it. It's a powerful weapon to have in your back pocket to fight AMD and a host of other diseases. Okra's got fiber, minerals, and vitamins (A, B complex, and C), not to mention antioxidants.

One 28-ounce can no salt added diced tomatoes

1 medium yellow onion, chopped

2 garlic cloves, minced

¼ pound okra, trimmed and sliced ½ inch thick (about 1 cup), or frozen cut okra, defrosted

½ teaspoon sea salt

¼ teaspoon freshly ground black pepper

In a medium saucepan, combine the tomatoes (undrained), onion, and garlic. Bring to a boil over high heat, then reduce the heat and simmer 10 minutes. Add the okra, salt, and pepper, and bring back to a boil, then reduce the heat to a simmer and cook until the okra is tender, about 15 to 20 minutes.

Nutritional Profile

Serving size: 1½ cups

Calories: 47

Protein: 2 g

Fiber: 3 g

Fat: less than 2 g

Saturated fat: less than 1 g

Sodium: 290 mg

Vitamin A: 1,181 IU

Vitamin C: 24 mg

Beta-carotene: 642 µg

Lutein and zeaxanthin: 157 µg

Lycopene: 3,242 µg

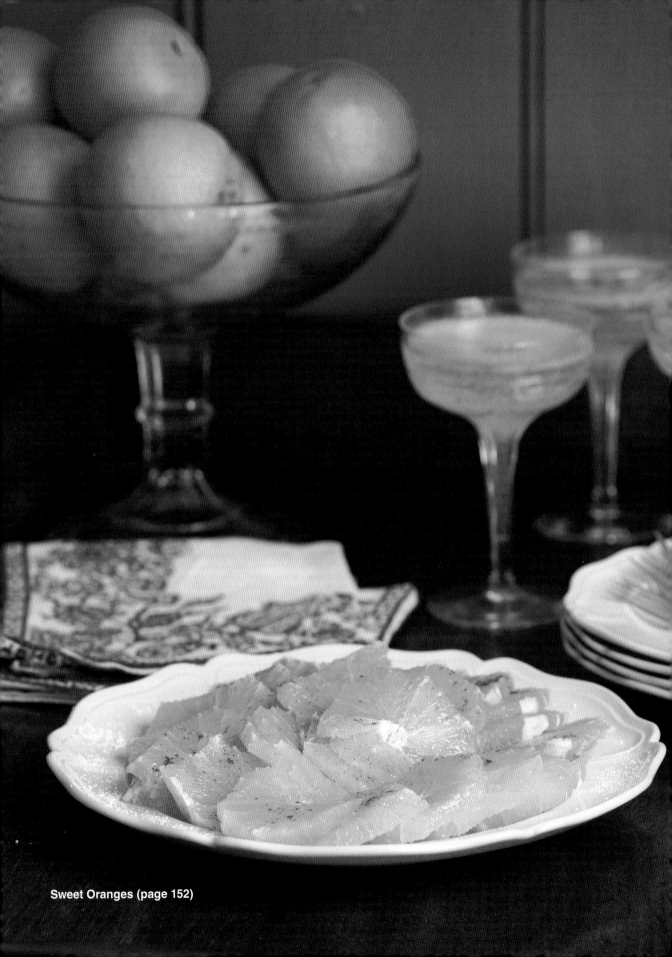

Sweet Oranges (page 152)

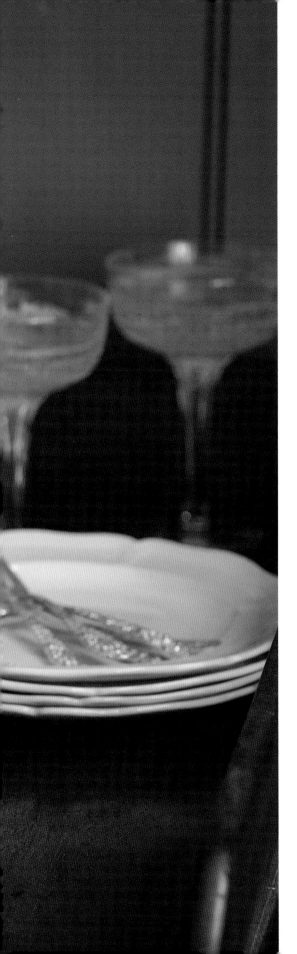

Desserts

Sweet Oranges

Strawberry Frozen Yogurt

Blueberry Frozen Yogurt

Mango Sorbet

Jody's Peach Soup

Peach Frozen Yogurt

Spiced Almonds with Cinnamon

Spa Baklava

Pear-Raspberry Galette

Carrot Cake

Chocolate-Beet Cupcakes with
    Chocolate-Yogurt Frosting

Sweet Oranges

SERVES 4

This simple dessert is vibrant, refreshing, and healthy. Vitamin C and beta-carotene are abundant in oranges.

- 4 navel oranges, peeled
- 2 tablespoons confectioners' sugar
- Cinnamon

Slice the oranges crosswise and arrange on individual plates. Dust with the sugar and cinnamon and serve immediately.

Nutritional Profile

Serving size: 1 orange

Calories: 84
Protein: 1 g
Fiber: 3 g
Fat: less than 1 g
Saturated fat: less than 1 g
Sodium: 1 mg
Vitamin A: 346 IU
Vitamin C: 83 mg
Beta-carotene: 122 µg
Lutein and zeaxanthin: 181 µg

"A man ought to carry himself in the world as an orange tree would if it could walk up and down in the garden, swinging perfume from every little censer it holds up to the air."

— *Henry Ward Beecher*

Strawberry Frozen Yogurt

SERVES 4

A low-calorie fruit, strawberries have nutritional zeal: they contain beta-carotene, vitamin A, and some lutein. The agave nectar that sweetens this dish can be found in most health food stores and some well-stocked supermarkets.

3	cups chopped strawberries
1⅓	cups low-fat plain yogurt
¼	cup agave nectar

Process all ingredients in a food processor until smooth. Pour into a 9 by 13-inch container and freeze, stirring every hour, until the mixture is firm around the edges and semifirm in the center, about 4 to 4 ½ hours. Return the mixture to a food processor and process until smooth. Serve immediately.

Nutritional Profile

Serving size: 1 cup

Calories: 128
Protein: 4 g
Fiber: 2 g
Fat: less than 1 g
Saturated fat: less than 1 g
Sodium: 46 mg
Vitamin A: 346 IU
Vitamin C: 68 mg
Vitamin D: 27 IU
Vitamin E: 2 IU
Beta-carotene: 8 µg
Lutein and zeaxanthin: 28 µg

Blueberry Frozen Yogurt

SERVES 4

Filled with vitamin C, dietary fiber, manganese, and antioxidants (especially anthocyanins, which give the fruit its blue hue), blueberries are dynamos. Indeed, regarding antioxidant activity, blueberries surpass most foods. Antioxidants help neutralize the unstable molecules (free radicals) that are linked to cancer, cardiovascular disease, macular degeneration, and other age-related diseases.

- 3 cups fresh blueberries
- 2 cups low-fat plain yogurt
- ½ cup sugar
- ¼ teaspoon pure vanilla extract

Process all ingredients in a food processor until smooth. Pour into a 9 by 13-inch container and freeze, stirring every hour, until the mixture is firm around the edges and semifirm in the center, about 4 to 4½ hours. Return the mixture to a food processor and process until smooth. Serve immediately.

Nutritional Profile

Serving size: ¾ cup

Calories: 158
Protein: 4 g
Fiber: 2 g
Fat: 1 g
Saturated fat: 1 g
Sodium: 58 mg
Vitamin A: 207 IU
Vitamin C: 8 mg
Vitamin E: 1 IU
Beta-carotene: 24 µg
Lutein and zeaxanthin: 59 µg

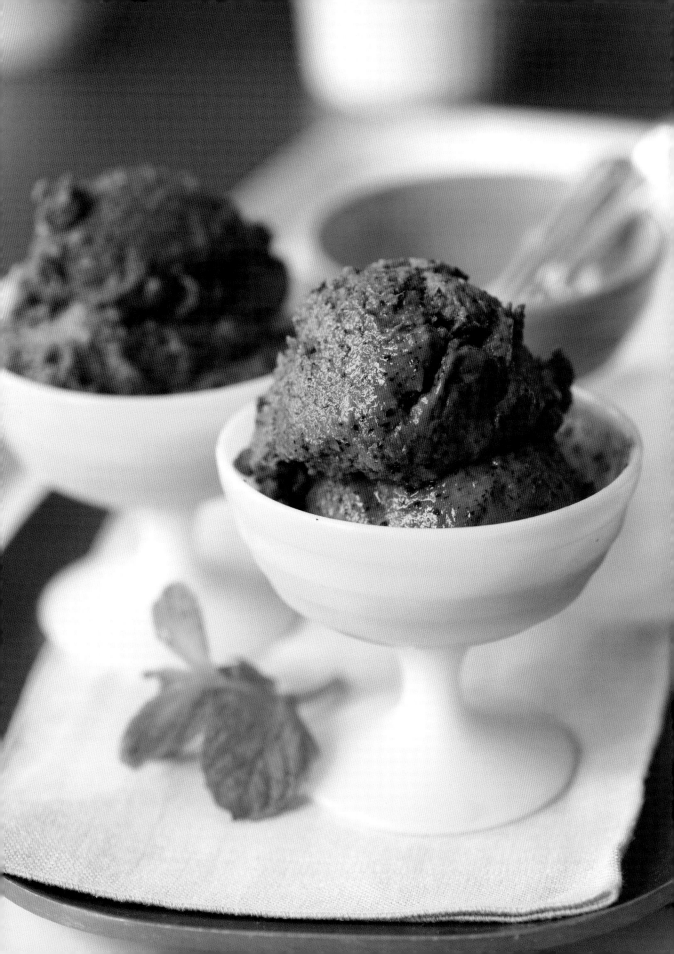

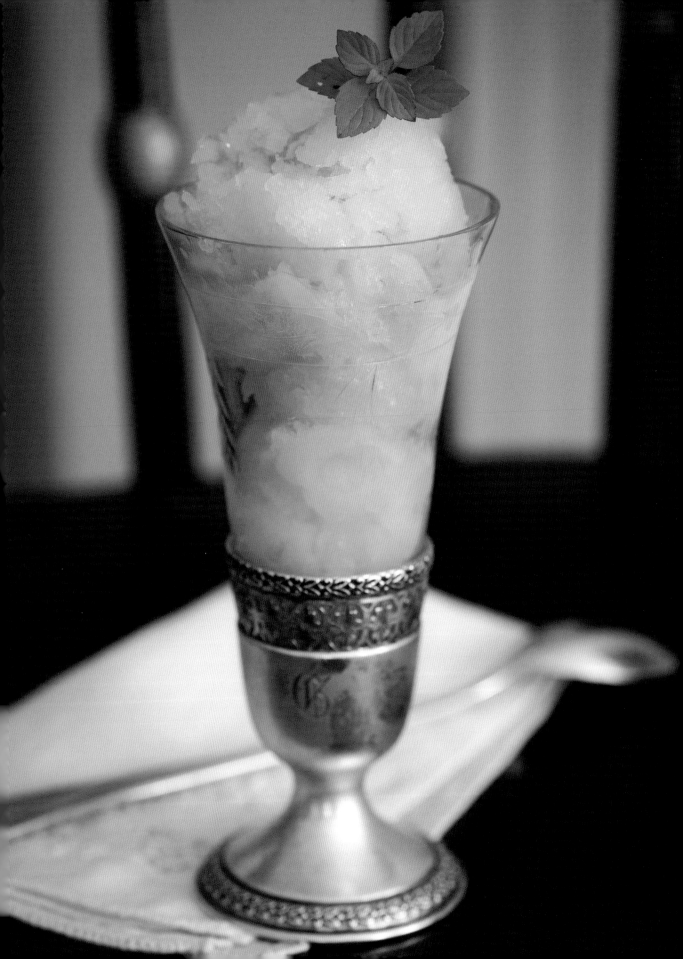

Mango Sorbet

SERVES 4–6

Similar in color to oranges, which are known for their high concentration of vitamin C, mangoes also have a good amount of vitamin A.

- 3 ripe mangoes, peeled, pitted, and coarsely chopped
  Juice of 1 lime
- 1 cup chilled simple syrup (see note below)
  Fresh mint, for garnish
  Fresh blueberries or pomegranate seeds, for garnish

Purée the mango in a food processor until smooth, then add the lime juice and syrup; and purée for a few pulses more. Transfer to a freezable container and freeze until firm and set, about 6 hours. When ready to serve, scoop the mango into bowls and garnish with mint and berries.

Note: To make simple syrup, combine 1 part water with 1 part sugar in a saucepan over high heat, stirring to dissolve the sugar. Bring to a boil, stirring occasionally, then remove from the heat and set aside to cool. When it's cool, chill the syrup in the refrigerator. Simple syrup will keep for several months in the refrigerator.

Nutritional Profile

Serving size: 1 cup

Calories: 239
Protein: 2 g
Fiber: 3 g
Fat: 1 g
Saturated fat: less than 1 g
Sodium: 4 mg
Vitamin A: 2,183 IU
Vitamin C: 74 mg
Vitamin E: 3 IU
Beta-carotene: 1,291 µg
Lutein and zeaxanthin: 46 µg
Lycopene: 6 µg

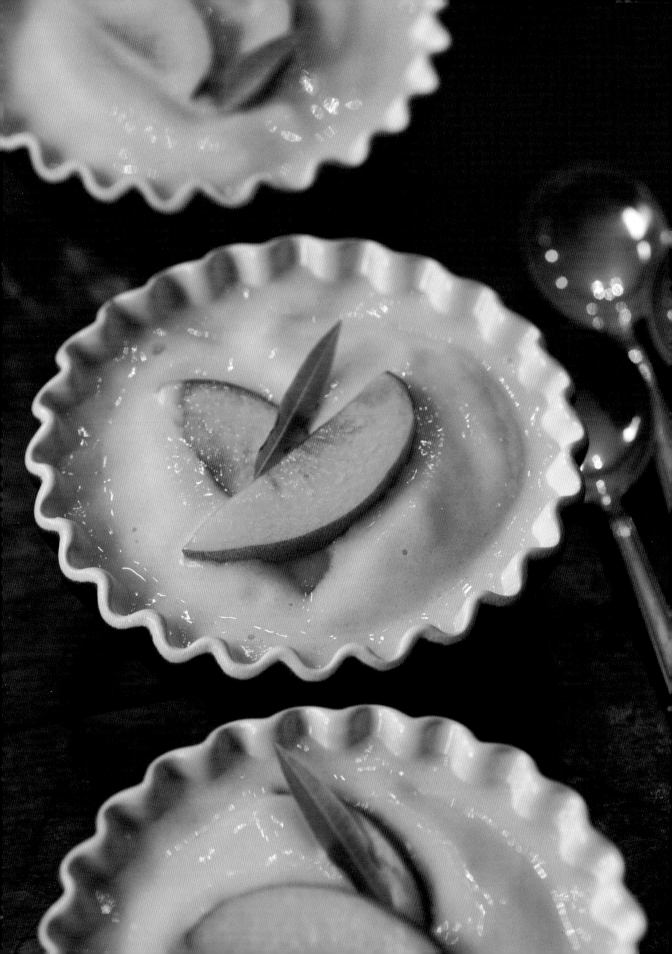

Jody's Peach Soup

This peach soup is simple, lovely, and tasty with a hefty helping of vitamins A and C. Garnish with fresh raspberries, sliced peaches, or a sprig of mint.

1 pound fresh or frozen peaches, pitted and halved (about 2 cups)

2 cups low-fat plain yogurt

1 tablespoon honey

1 tablespoon freshly squeezed lemon juice

Combine the ingredients in a blender and purée until smooth. Serve cold. Garnish with fresh fruit or a mint sprig.

Nutritional Profile

Serving size: 1 cup

Calories: 110

Protein: 5 g

Fiber: 1 g

Fat: 2 g

Saturated fat: 1 g

Sodium: 68 mg

Vitamin A: 385 IU

Vitamin C: 8 mg

Lutein and zeaxanthin: less than 1 µg

"A Georgia peach, a real Georgia peach, a backyard great-grandmother's orchard peach, is as thickly furred as a sweater, and so fluent and sweet that once you bite through the flannel, it brings tears to your eyes." — *Melissa Fay Greene*

Peach Frozen Yogurt

SERVES 4–6

Succulent and beautiful, peaches have certain phytochemicals that may inhibit cancerous tumors and are high in iron and potassium.

1	pound fresh peaches, pitted and halved (about 2 cups)
One	6-ounce container nonfat plain yogurt
¼	cup agave nectar
2	teaspoons flaxseed oil
½	teaspoon pure vanilla extract

Process all ingredients in a food processor until smooth. Pour into a 9 by 13-inch container and freeze, stirring every hour, until the mixture is firm around the edges and semifirm in the center, about 4 to 4½ hours. Return the mixture to a food processor and process until smooth. Serve immediately.

Nutritional Profile

Serving size: 1 cup

Calories: 117
Protein: 2 g
Fiber: 1 g
Fat: 2 g
Saturated fat: less than 1 g
Sodium: 20 mg
Vitamin A: 335 IU
Vitamin C: 7 mg
Vitamin D: 12 IU
Vitamin E: 1 IU
Omega-3 fatty acids: 1 g

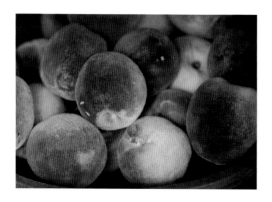

Spiced Almonds
with Cinnamon

MAKES 2 CUPS

We're nuts about almonds. A handful of almonds (20 nuts) gives you 40 percent of your daily vitamin E allowance (6 mg of vitamin E), and there's more magnesium found in them than in spinach. Just be aware of the number eaten at one time, since nuts are also high in calories.

1	large egg white
⅓	cup sugar
2	teaspoons ground cardamom
1	teaspoon ground cinnamon
½	teaspoon ground allspice
¼	teaspoon sea salt
¼	teaspoon freshly grated nutmeg
2	cups raw whole almonds

Nutritional Profile

Serving size: ¼ cup

Calories: 243
Protein: 8 g
Fiber: 5 g
Fat: 18 g
Saturated fat: 1 g
Sodium: 95 mg
Vitamin A: 2 IU
Vitamin E: 14 IU
Zinc: 1 mg
Beta-carotene: 1 µg
Lutein and zeaxanthin: 1 µg

Preheat the oven to 350°F. Spray a rimmed baking sheet with nonstick cooking spray. Set aside.

Beat the egg white in a medium bowl until frothy but not stiff. In a separate bowl, combine all the remaining ingredients except the almonds. Toss the almonds in the egg white and then into the spice mix, stirring to blend.

Spread in a single layer on the prepared baking sheet and bake for 15 to 20 minutes, stirring after 10 minutes, until toasted and fragrant. Remove to a rack to cool slightly. Store in an airtight container up to a week.

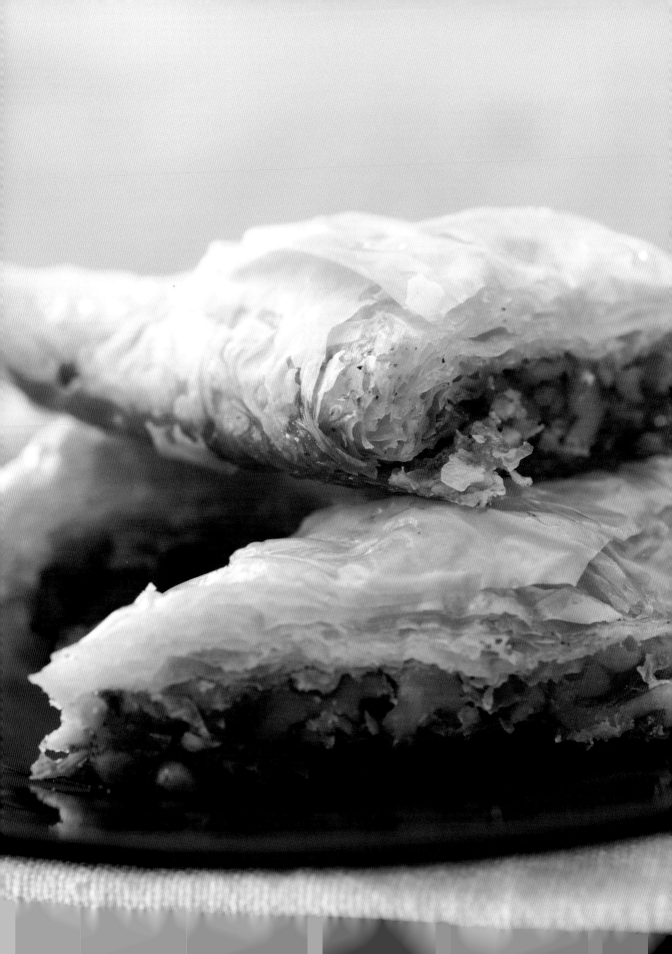

Spa Baklava

SERVES 12

Is healthy dessert an oxymoron? It needn't be; this baklava from Canyon Ranch is light and delicious, with walnuts providing linolenic acid, a type of omega-3.

- ½ cup walnuts, chopped
- 1 tablespoon granulated sugar
- ¼ teaspoon ground cinnamon
- ¼ teaspoon ground cloves
- 2 tablespoons unsalted butter, melted
- 2 tablespoons canola oil
- 8 sheets phyllo dough, cut in half

LEMON SIMPLE SYRUP

- ½ cup sugar
- ¼ cup water
- ¼ teaspoon grated lemon zest
- ½ tablespoon fresh lemon juice
- ¼ cinnamon stick

Combine the walnuts, sugar, cinnamon, and cloves in a small bowl. Set it aside.

In another bowl, combine the melted butter and oil.

CONTINUED

Unfold the phyllo sheets and cover them with plastic to keep moist. Lightly spray the bottom of a 9 by 9-inch square baking pan or cookie sheet with nonstick cooking spray.

Lightly brush 4 sheets of phyllo with the butter mixture. Lay them in the pan, allowing them to fold upward at the sides of the pan, if necessary. Top with half of the nut mixture. Brush 4 more phyllo sheets with the butter mixture and lay them over the nut mixture. Spread the remaining nut mixture over the phyllo sheets. Brush the remaining sheets with the butter mixture and place them over the nut mixture, folding the sides of the phyllo inward when necessary.

Chill until the butter is hardened. Score the baklava diagonally to make 12 triangles.

Preheat the oven to 350°F. Bake for 35 to 40 minutes or until golden brown.

In a small sauté pan, combine the ingredients for the simple syrup and bring to a boil. Simmer until the sugar is dissolved. Pour the mixture evenly over the baked baklava. Cool and slice.

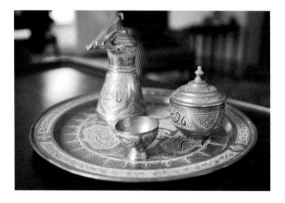

Nutritional Profile

Serving size: 1 triangle

Calories: 144
Protein: 2 g
Fiber: 1 g
Fat: 8 g
Saturated fat: 2 g
Sodium: 62 mg
Vitamin A: 60 IU
Vitamin D: 1 IU
Vitamin E: 1 IU
Beta-carotene: 5 µg
Lutein and zeaxanthin: 2 µg
Omega-3 fatty acids: 1 g

Pear-Raspberry Galette

SERVES 8–10

This rustic yet sophisticated dessert is by Catrine Kelty, a talented French food stylist who worked on this book. Raspberries contain minerals and vitamins that promote eye health, while pears protect you from free radicals and encourage cardiovascular health. Several servings of fruit daily might lower your risk of age-related macular degeneration.

DOUGH

- 1 cup whole wheat pastry flour (not whole wheat flour)
- 2 tablespoons sugar
- ¼ teaspoon sea salt
- 1 teaspoon ground cinnamon
- ½ cup unsalted butter (1 stick), chilled, cut into small pieces
- 3 to 4 tablespoons ice-cold water

FOR THE FILLING

- 3 tablespoons all-purpose flour
- 1 tablespoon sugar
- 1 tablespoon freshly grated lemon zest
- ½ teaspoon ground cinnamon
- ¼ teaspoon freshly grated nutmeg
- Pinch of sea salt
- 1 pound (about 2 large) ripe but still firm Bartlett or Anjou pears, peeled, cored, and sliced ¼ inch thick
- 1 pint fresh raspberries
- ¼ cup (4 tablespoons) unsalted butter, chilled and cut into small pieces
- Juice of ½ lemon

CONTINUED

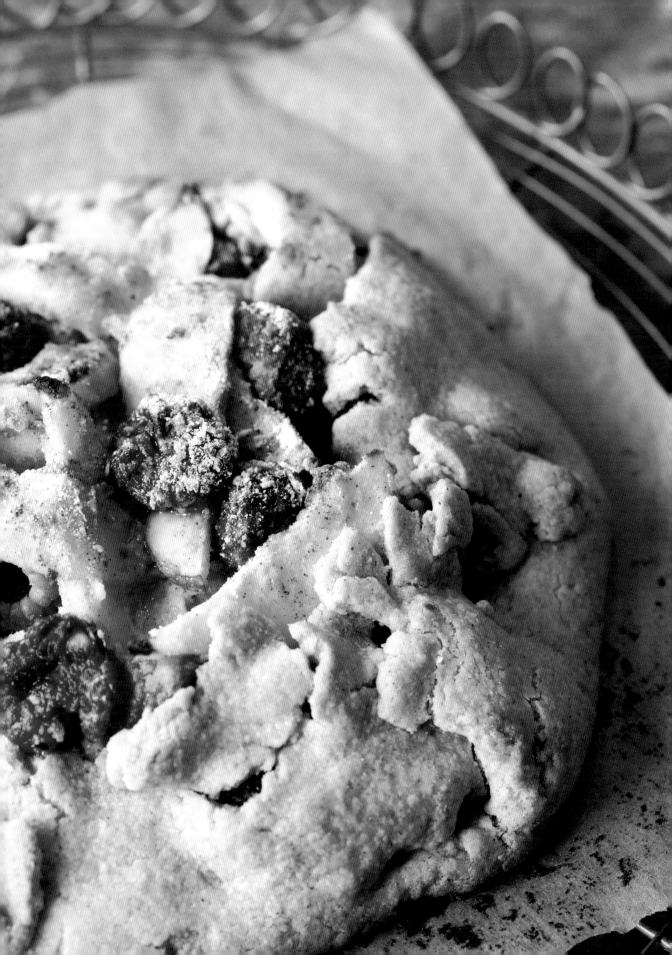

In the bowl of a food processor, mix the pastry flour, sugar, salt, and cinnamon. Pulse to combine. Sprinkle the butter on the dry ingredients and pulse until it looks like oatmeal (about 3 pulses of 15 seconds each). With the motor running, add 3 tablespoons of water, and 1 additional tablespoon if the dough seems too dry.

When the dough is combined, transfer it to a clean surface and knead a few times (taking care not to overwork the dough) until it comes together. Shape it into a disk, wrap it in plastic, and let it rest at least 1 hour in the refrigerator.

When you're ready to make the galette, take the dough out of the refrigerator to warm it slightly. Mix the all-purpose flour, sugar, lemon zest, cinnamon, nutmeg, and salt in a bowl. Very gently mix in the pears, raspberries, and butter, making sure they are all coated with the flour mixture but still intact. Sprinkle with the lemon juice and stir to combine.

On a piece of parchment paper, roll out the dough to a 10- to 12-inch circle, about ¼ inch thick. Cover the dough with the filling, making sure to distribute the raspberries and butter evenly, leaving a 2-inch border. Gently fold the border over the mixture, pleating it to create a circle.

Transfer the parchment to a baking sheet and refrigerate the galette for at least 15 minutes. In the meantime, preheat the oven to 450°F. Bake the galette for 20 to 25 minutes, until the crust is golden and the filling is tender and bubbles slightly. Serve warm or at room temperature.

Nutritional Profile

Serving size: 1 slice

Calories: 392

Protein: 2 g

Fiber: 6 g

Fat: 31 g

Saturated fat: 19 g

Sodium: 155 mg

Vitamin A: 969 IU

Vitamin C: 11 mg

Vitamin D: 23 IU

Vitamin E: 2 IU

Beta-carotene: 70 µg

Lutein and zeaxanthin: 62 µg

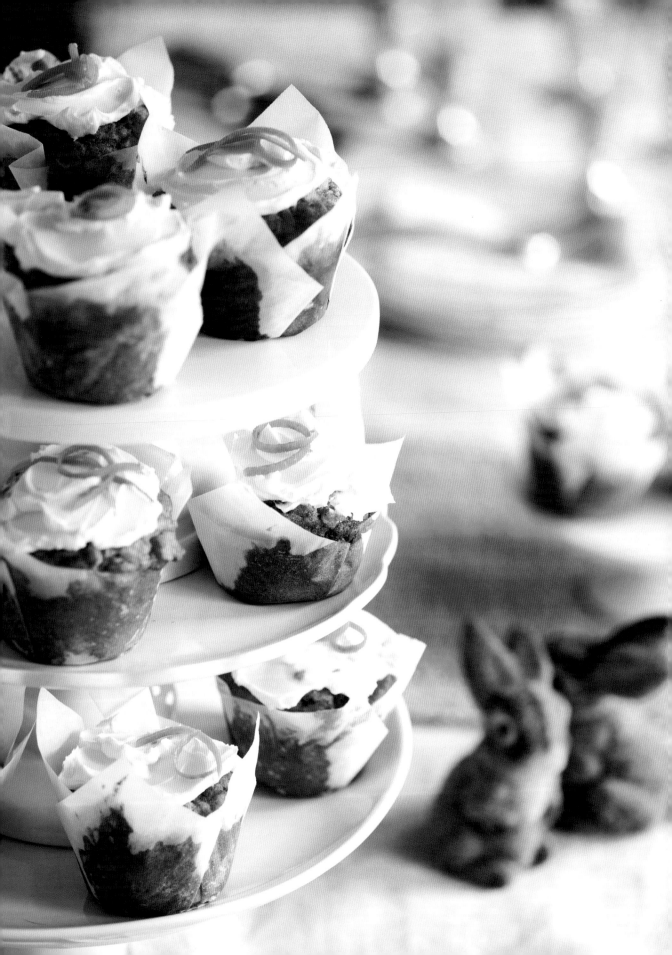

Carrot Cake

MAKES 1 CAKE | 16 SERVINGS

Before World War II, the English were not huge eaters of carrots, which posed a problem when there was a glut of carrots during the war. Leveraging the belief that carotene helps night vision, the British government promoted carrots with slogans such as "Carrots keep you healthy and help you see in the blackout." Tons of dehydrated carrots were shipped to soldiers overseas in containers to prevent the loss of carotene, and the government claimed that carrots were largely responsible for RAF successes in shooting down Luftwaffe planes. This campaign reduced the carrot surplus and made for a healthier nation when food supplies were scarce.

FOR THE CAKE

Unsalted butter, for greasing pans

2 cups whole wheat pastry flour, plus more for the cake pans

2 teaspoons baking soda

¼ teaspoon sea salt

1 tablespoon ground cinnamon

3 large eggs

1 cup low-fat milk

½ cup firmly packed brown sugar

½ cup canola oil

2 teaspoons pure vanilla extract

One 8-ounce can (1 cup) crushed pineapple with juice

1 pound carrots, grated (about 2 cups)

¼ cup unsweetened coconut flakes

¼ cup chopped walnuts

¼ cup currants

CONTINUED

  12 ounces reduced-fat cream cheese, room temperature

  ⅓ cup confectioners' sugar

  2 tablespoons orange juice

  1 teaspoon pure vanilla extract

      Freshly grated nutmeg, for dusting

Preheat the oven to 350°F. Butter and flour two round cake pans. Set aside.

In a medium bowl, combine the 2 cups of flour, baking soda, salt, and cinnamon. In a large bowl, whisk together the eggs, milk, brown sugar, oil, and vanilla. Stir in the pineapple, carrots, and coconut. Add the dry ingredients and mix to combine. Add the walnuts and currants and spoon the mixture evenly into the cake pans. Bake 40 to 45 minutes, until a toothpick comes out clean. Transfer the cakes to a rack to cool.

To make the frosting, whisk the cream cheese, confectioners' sugar, orange juice, and vanilla in a medium bowl. To assemble the cake, place one layer flat side up on a plate and cover the top with frosting. Place the second layer flat side down on top of the first layer and spread the frosting over the top and sides. Dust with nutmeg.

Nutritional Profile

Serving size: 1 slice

Calories: 264

Protein: 6 g

Fiber: 4 g

Fat: 14 g

Saturated fat: 4 g

Sodium: 344 mg

Vitamin A: 4,935 IU

Vitamin C: 7 mg

Vitamin D: 10 IU

Vitamin E: 2 IU

Beta-carotene: 2,356 µg

Lutein and zeaxanthin: 123 µg

Omega-3 fatty acids: 1 g

Chocolate-Beet Cupcakes with Chocolate-Yogurt Frosting

MAKES 18 CUPCAKES

Beets with chocolate? Deceptively delicious, the beets add fiber and carotenoids. These dark-chocolate cakes are so satisfying, you won't believe the intense flavor comes from cocoa powder and the grated root vegetable.

2	cups all-purpose flour
½	cup cocoa powder
1	teaspoon baking soda
1	teaspoon baking powder
½	teaspoon salt
3	large eggs, beaten
1	cup vegetable oil
1½	cups sugar
2	teaspoons pure vanilla extract
2	cups grated cooked beets (from 3 to 4 medium beets, boiled, cooled, peeled, and grated or pulse-chopped in a food processor)

Preheat the oven to 350°F and line 18 cups in two muffin pans with paper liners (or bake in two batches). In a small bowl, combine the flour, cocoa powder, baking soda, baking powder, and salt. Set aside.

In a mixing bowl, combine the eggs, oil, and sugar and beat until smooth. Beat in the vanilla. Beat in the dry ingredients in two additions until just combined; stir in the beets. Spoon into the paper-lined muffin cups, filling three-quarters full. Bake until the cupcakes bounce back when touched lightly in the center, 25 to 30 minutes. Cool the cupcakes completely, then frost with Chocolate-Yogurt Frosting.

CONTINUED

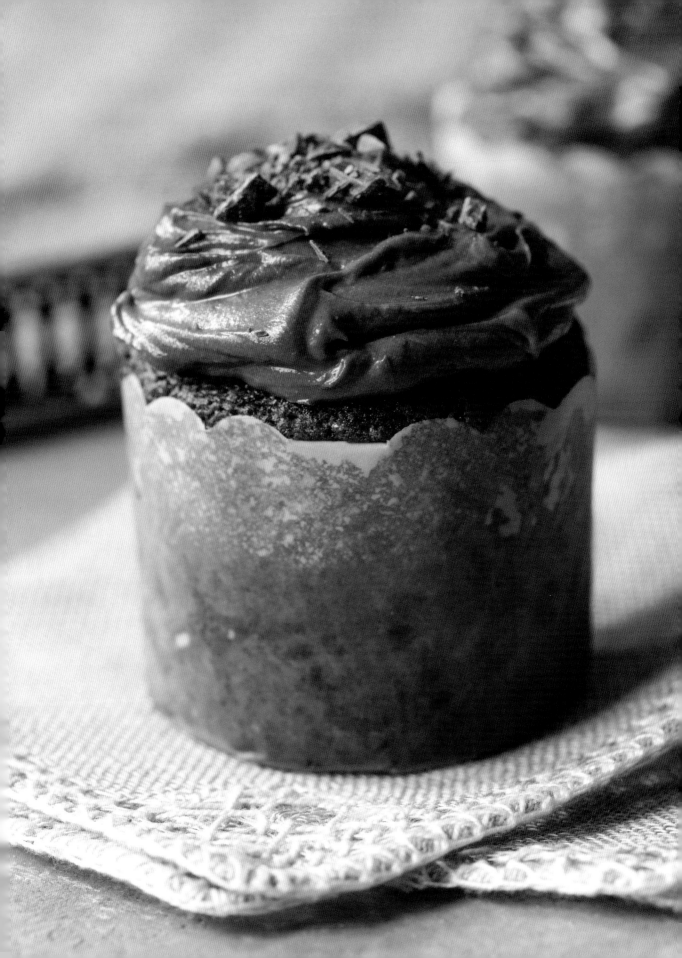

Chocolate-Yogurt Frosting

Before the two ingredients in this recipe are combined, it's important that both the melted chocolate and the yogurt are as close to room temperature as possible.

1½ cups semisweet chocolate chips

1½ cups raspberry Greek yogurt, room temperature

Place the chocolate chips in a microwave-safe bowl. Heat in the microwave at 50 percent power at 30-second intervals, stirring every 30 seconds, until the chocolate is melted and smooth. Allow it to cool to room temperature. Stir in the yogurt 1 large spoonful at a time, stirring until the frosting is smooth. (If the frosting gets too stiff, allow it to rest until it is spreadable.)

Tip: To make frosting even easier, chill the cupcakes first until they're firm to the touch.

Nutritional Profile

Serving size: 1 cupcake

Calories: 330
Protein: 5 g
Fiber: 2 g
Fat: 18 g
Saturated fat: 4 g
Sodium: 376 mg
Vitamin A: 51 IU
Vitamin C: 1 mg
Vitamin D: 7 IU
Vitamin E: 4 IU
Beta-carotene: 3.64 µg
Lutein and zeaxanthin: 47 µg

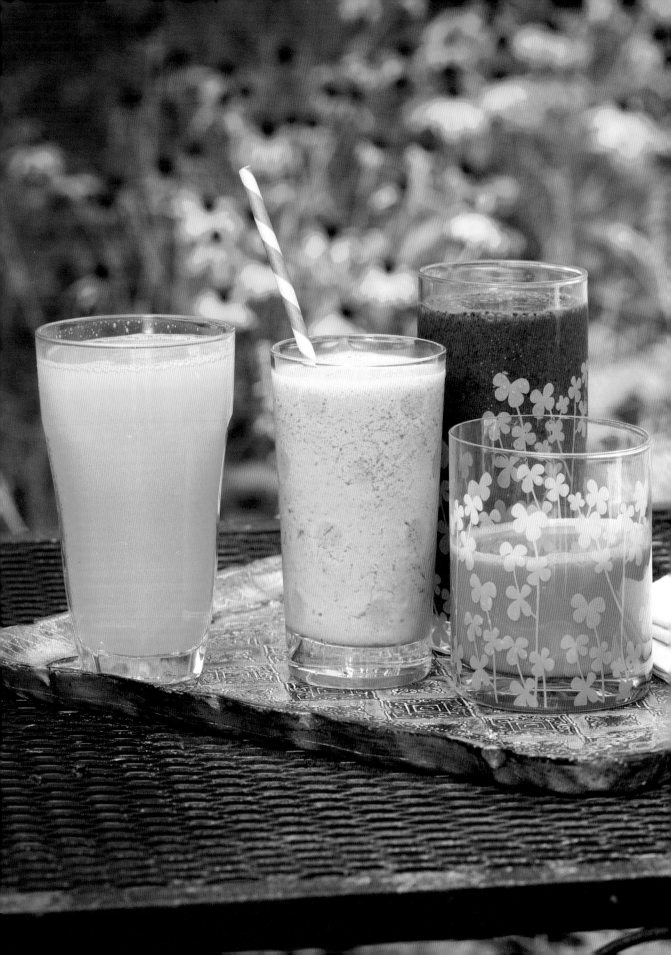

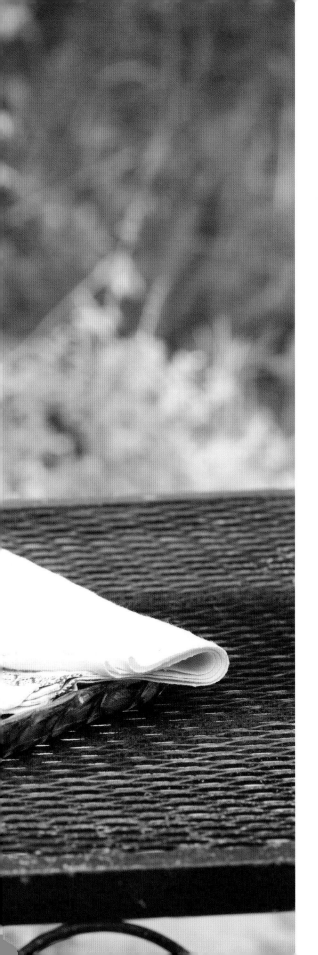

Healthy Drinks

Banana-Blueberry-
  Pomegranate Smoothie

Kale-Banana Smoothie

Blueberry Smoothie

Power Juice

Cucumber-Kale Drink

Orange-Grapefruit Juice

Carrot-Ginger Juice

Strawberry-Orange Smoothie

Watermelon-Citrus Cooler

Apple-Celery Juice

Red Pepper Juice

Homemade Vegetable Juice

Banana-Blueberry-Pomegranate Smoothie

SERVES 2

This drink sneaks in a lot of bang for the buck—carotenoids from the kale, lutein from the blueberries, vitamin C from the pomegranate juice, and potassium from the bananas, plus fiber.

1 ripe banana

2 kale leaves, stems removed

1 cup blueberries

2 cups pomegranate juice

1 tablespoon freshly squeezed lime juice

Combine all the ingredients in a blender and purée until smooth, about 45 to 60 seconds. Chill briefly if desired. Serve immediately.

Nutritional Profile

Serving Size: 2 cups

Calories: 262

Protein: 4 g

Fiber: 5 g

Fat: 1 g

Saturated fat: less than 1 g

Sodium: 33 mg

Vitamin A: 7,808 IU

Vitamin C: 135 mg

Vitamin E: 2 IU

Zinc: 1 mg

Beta-carotene: 4,677 µg

Lutein and zeaxanthin: 19,946 µg

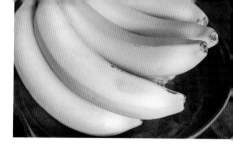

Kale-Banana Smoothie

SERVES 2

There's a lot shaking in this smoothie—an abundance of nutrients and contrasting flavors, which makes for a worthy drink.

- 1 cup chopped green kale, stems removed
- 1 large stalk celery, coarsely chopped
- 1 ripe banana
- ½ cup apple juice
- ¼ cup water
- ½ cup ice
- 1 tablespoon freshly squeezed lime juice
- 1 teaspoon wheat germ (or ground flaxseeds or oat/rice bran)

Combine all the ingredients in a blender and purée until smooth, about 45 to 60 seconds. Chill briefly or serve immediately.

Nutritional Profile

Serving Size: 2 cups

Calories: 101
Protein: 2 g
Fiber: 3 g
Fat: 1 g
Saturated fat: less than 1 g
Sodium: 45 mg
Vitamin A: 5,331 IU
Vitamin C: 48 mg
Vitamin E: 1 IU
Beta-carotene: 3,193 µg
Lutein and zeaxanthin: 13,351 µg

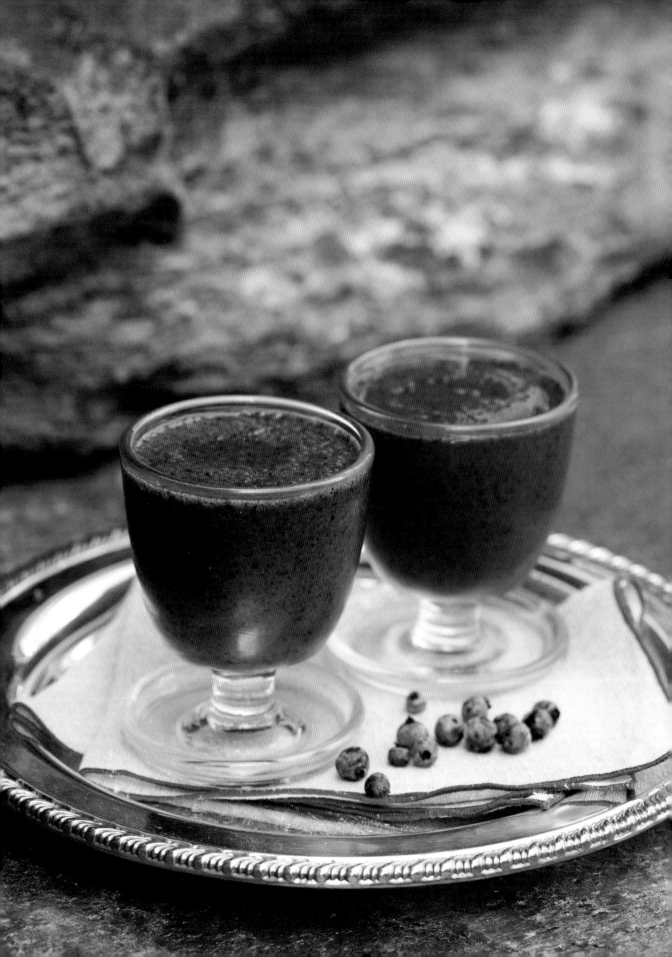

Blueberry Smoothie

SERVES 2

With some of the highest antioxidant protection of all fruits, blueberries are also a source of vitamin A, folate, and potassium.

1   cup frozen blueberries
1   cup vanilla soymilk
½   ripe banana
1   tablespoon flaxseed oil

Combine all the ingredients in a blender and purée until smooth, about 45 to 60 seconds. Chill briefly if desired. Serve immediately.

"I may never be happy, but tonight I am content. Nothing more than an empty house, the warm hazy weariness from a day spent setting strawberry runners in the sun, a glass of cool sweet milk, and a shallow dish of blueberries bathed in cream."

— *Sylvia Plath*

Nutritional Profile

Serving Size: 1 cup

Calories: 172
Protein: 4 g
Fiber: 3 g
Fat: 9 g
Saturated fat: 1 g
Sodium: 48 mg
Vitamin A: 272 IU
Vitamin C: 4 mg
Vitamin D: 60 IU
Beta-carotene: 8 µg
Lutein and zeaxanthin: 6 µg
Omega-3 fatty acids: 4 g

Power Juice

SERVES 2

With an earthy, almost grassy flavor that is balanced by the sweetness of the carrots, this is an eye-healthy pick-me-up in the afternoon.

1   cup spinach, stems removed
2   celery stalks with leaves
2   carrots, peeled
1   Granny Smith apple, cored

Combine all the ingredients in a juicer and serve.

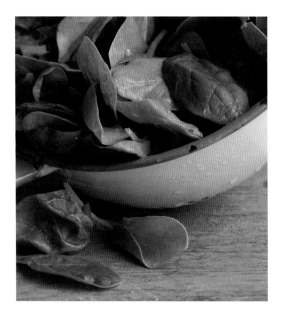

Nutritional Profile

Serving size: ¾ cup

Calories: 78
Protein: 2 g
Fiber: 5 g
Fat: less than 1 g
Saturated fat: less than 1 g
Sodium: 94 mg
Vitamin A: 13,655 IU
Vitamin C: 13 mg
Vitamin E: 2 IU
Beta-carotene: 6,937 µg
Lutein and zeaxanthin: 2,149 µg
Lycopene: 1 µg

Cucumber-Kale Drink

SERVES 2

Kale for what ails you. A pretty forest green, this herbal grassy beverage tastes like you are drinking good health, and you are—with macular degeneration a leading cause of legal blindness in people over age 55, it's a drink to your health.

3 cups loosely chopped kale, stems removed

¾ cup chopped pineapple (fresh or canned)

1 large organic cucumber, skin left on

1 small apple, cored and peeled

2 teaspoons freshly squeezed lemon juice

½ teaspoon minced fresh ginger

½ cup fresh mint leaves, stems removed

1 tablespoon flaxseed oil

Combine all the ingredients in a juicer and serve.

Nutritional Profile

Serving Size: 2 cups

Calories: 210

Protein: 6 g

Fiber: 7 g

Fat: 8 g

Saturated fat: 1 g

Sodium: 47 mg

Vitamin A: 16,104 IU

Vitamin C: 167 mg

Zinc: 1 mg

Beta-carotene: 9,496 µg

Lutein and zeaxanthin: 39,770 µg

Omega-3 fatty acids: 4 g

Orange-Grapefruit Juice

SERVES 2

While all grapefruits contain vitamin C and folate, pink and red grapefruits are excellent sources of carotenoids as well.

3 oranges

1 pink grapefruit

Lightly roll the fruit on the counter, then cut each in half. Use a citrus reamer or hand juicer to squeeze into a container. Stir and pour into glasses.

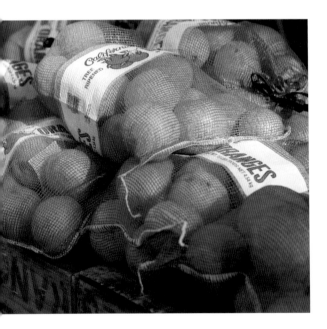

Nutritional Profile

Serving Size: 2 cups

Calories: 156

Protein: 3 g

Fiber: 6 g

Fat: less than 1 g

Saturated fat: less than 1 g

Sodium: 2 mg

Vitamin A: 2,057 IU

Vitamin C: 181 mg

Beta-carotene: 1,099 µg

Lutein and zeaxanthin: 281 µg

Lycopene: 1,884 µg

Carrot-Ginger Juice

SERVES 2

Eight ounces of carrot juice yield as much as 20 percent of your recommended daily requirement of vitamin C and a high dose of beta-carotene and vitamin A.

- 8 large organic peeled carrots, coarsely chopped
- ¼ teaspoon minced fresh ginger
- 2 teaspoons freshly squeezed lemon juice
- 2 cups boiling water

Combine all the ingredients in a blender and blend for 2 minutes. Strain through a fine-mesh sieve. Chill before serving.

Nutritional Profile

Serving Size: 2 cups

Calories: 120
Protein: 3 g
Fiber: 8 g
Fat: 1 g
Saturated fat: less than 1 g
Sodium: 208 mg
Vitamin A: 48,114 IU
Vitamin C: 19 mg
Vitamin E: 3 IU
Zinc: 1 mg
Beta-carotene: 23,860 µg
Lutein and zeaxanthin: 738 µg
Lycopene: 3 µg

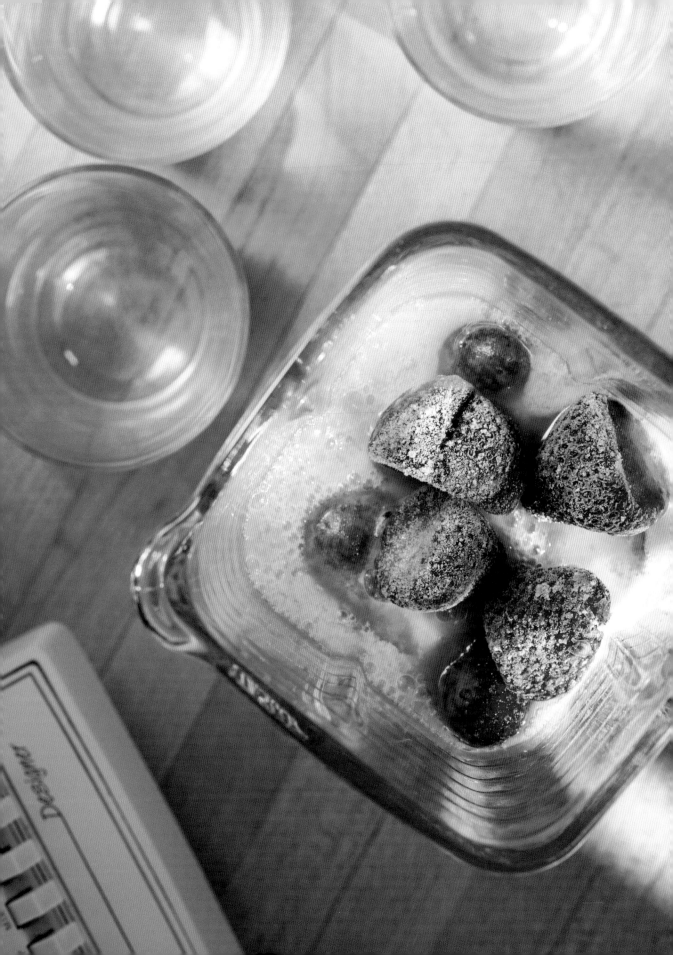

Strawberry-Orange Smoothie

SERVES 2

Oranges are a nutritious source of vitamin C and potassium.

- 1 cup frozen strawberries
- 1 cup orange juice
- 1 cup soymilk

Combine all the ingredients in a blender and purée until smooth, about 45 to 60 seconds. Serve immediately.

Nutritional Profile

Serving Size: 1 cup

Calories: 155

Protein: 5 g

Fiber: 2 g

Fat: 2 g

Saturated fat: less than 1 g

Sodium: 64 mg

Vitamin A: 58 IU

Vitamin C: 46 mg

Beta-carotene: 11 µg

Lutein and zeaxanthin: 36 µg

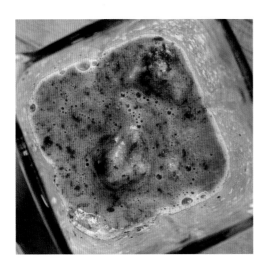

Watermelon-Citrus Cooler

SERVES 4

What could be more cooling than a slice of watermelon? A glass of it. Turn it into a cocktail by adding a splash of rum and a dusting of confectioners' sugar—and feel good about the vitamin A and beta-carotene in each glass.

1 tangerine, peeled, seeded, and quartered

4 cups chilled cubed watermelon, seeds removed (or choose a seedless melon)

Juice of ½ lime

2 teaspoons freshly chopped fresh mint leaves

Combine all the ingredients in a blender and purée until smooth, about 45 to 60 seconds. Serve immediately.

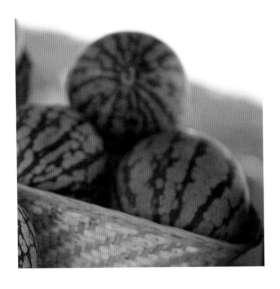

Nutritional Profile

Serving Size: 2 cups

Calories: 55

Protein: 1 g

Fiber: 2 g

Fat: less than 1 g

Saturated fat: less than 1 g

Sodium: 8 mg

Vitamin A: 697 IU

Vitamin C: 15 mg

Beta-carotene: 362 µg

Lutein and zeaxanthin: 30 µg

Apple-Celery Juice

SERVES 2

They weren't kidding when they said an apple a day; preliminary research indicates that apples may benefit those with macular degeneration, not to mention decreasing the risk for other issues from asthma to lung cancer. This juice is also good on ice with a shot of vodka.

2   Granny Smith apples, seeded and coarsely chopped

4   McIntosh apples, seeded and coarsely chopped

2   celery stalks, chopped

Combine all the ingredients in a blender and blend for 1 minute. Strain through a fine-mesh sieve and serve.

Nutritional Profile

Serving Size: 2 cups

Calories: 216

Protein: 2 g

Fiber: 15 g

Fat: 1 g

Saturated fat: less than 1 g

Sodium: 38 mg

Vitamin A: 501 IU

Vitamin C: 29 mg

Vitamin E: 2 IU

Beta-carotene: 269 µg

Lutein and zeaxanthin: 286 µg

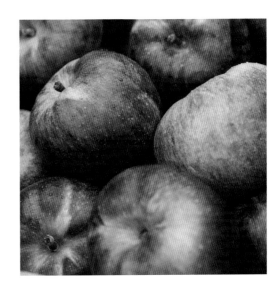

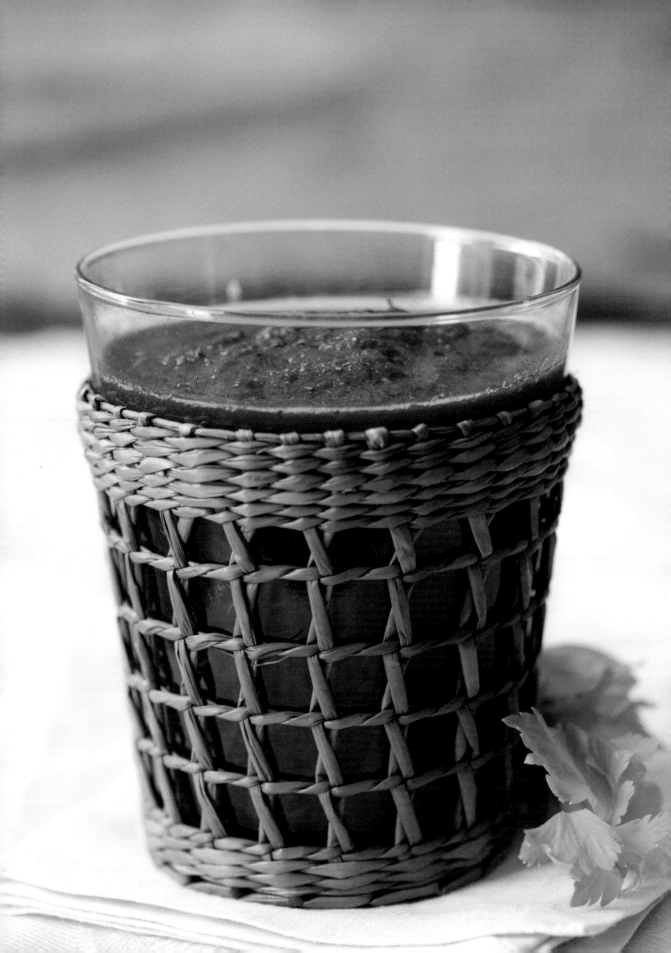

Red Pepper Juice

SERVES 3

U nwaxed red bell peppers can be found at health food stores. Look for perfect peppers with no blemishes and a taut, shiny skin. The pigment that turns their skin red (or yellow or orange) is good for you.

  6 unwaxed red bell peppers, cored, seeded, and coarsely chopped

     Juice of 1 lemon

     Sea salt and freshly ground black pepper, to taste

Combine all the ingredients in a blender and blend for 1 minute. Strain through a fine-mesh sieve and serve.

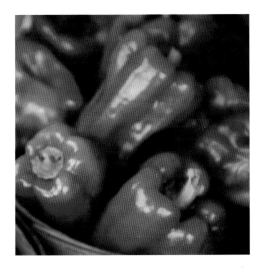

Nutritional Profile

Serving size: ⅔ cup

Calories: 49

Protein: 2 g

Fiber: 3 g

Sodium: 239 mg

Vitamin A: 4,636 IU

Vitamin C: 193 mg

Vitamin E: 4 IU

Beta-carotene: 2,404 µg

Lutein and zeaxanthin: 78 µg

Homemade Vegetable Juice

The benefits of making your own vegetable juice are many—you can customize the ingredients, select only the freshest vegetables, and avoid the sodium found in canned juices.

- 6 carrots, chopped
- 3 celery stalks, chopped
- 6 large tomatoes, cored and quartered
- 1 red bell pepper, cored, seeded, and chopped
- 1 green bell pepper, cored, seeded, and chopped
- 1 small white onion, halved
- 1 fresh beet, peeled and cut into eighths
- 2 cups fresh spinach
  Small handful fresh parsley
- 2 garlic cloves, chopped
  Freshly ground black pepper, to taste
  Juice of 2 lemons
- 2 teaspoons prepared horseradish

In a large soup pot, bring the carrots, celery, tomatoes, red and green bell peppers, onion, beet, and 1 cup of water to a boil, then simmer until the vegetables are soft, about 30 minutes. Combine all the ingredients in a blender or food processor and blend for 1½ minutes. If the juice is too thick, add a little more water. Chill before serving.

Nutritional Profile

Serving Size: 1 cup

Calories: 57

Protein: 2 g

Fiber: 4 g

Fat: 1 g

Sodium: 69 mg

Vitamin A: 9,169 IU

Vitamin C: 48 mg

Vitamin E: 2 IU

Beta-carotene: 4,663 µg

Lutein and zeaxanthin: 1,062 µg

Lycopene: 2,810 µg

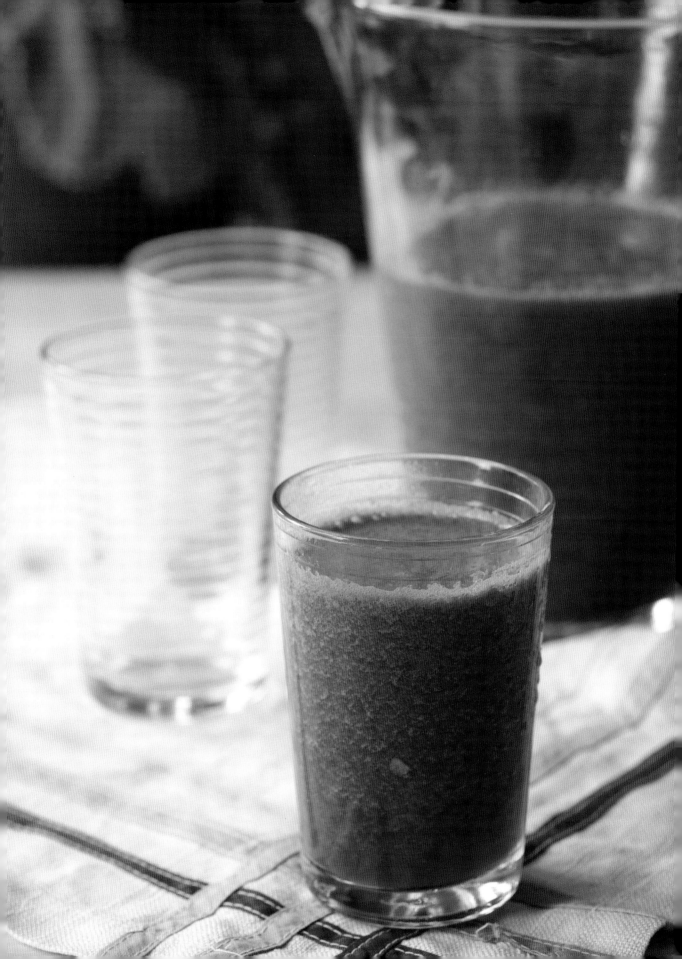

About the Authors

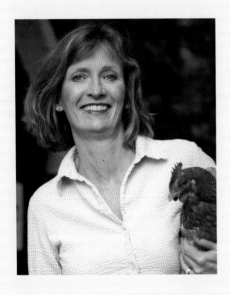

Jennifer Trainer Thompson is the author or coauthor of 16 books ranging in subjects from nuclear power to cooking. Nominated for three James Beard Awards, she has written numerous cookbooks, including *The Fresh Egg Cookbook, Hot Sauce!, The Yachting Cookbook,* and *Jump Up & Kiss Me: Spicy Vegetarian Cooking*. She is the chef and creator of the all-natural line of spicy sauces called Jump Up & Kiss Me, and a leader in the spicy foods movement. She is the coauthor of *Nuclear Power: Both Sides* and *Beyond Einstein: The Cosmic Quest for the Theory of the Universe*, both of which presented complicated scientific topics to the layman. A journalist for over 20 years, Jennifer has also written about topics that interest her—science, food, travel, art, and lifestyle—for *The New York Times, Travel + Leisure, Omni, Discover, Harvard Magazine,* and on her blog, jumpupandkiss.me.

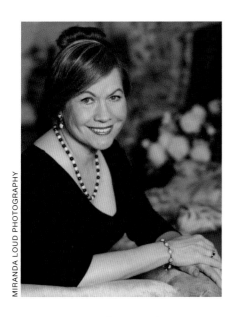

Johanna M. Seddon, MD, ScM, is a renowned macular degeneration clinician, researcher, author, and genetic epidemiologist. A professor of ophthalmology at Tufts University School of Medicine, she is the Founding Director of the Ophthalmic Epidemiology and Genetics Service at the New England Eye Center, Tufts Medical Center in Boston, Massachusetts. Her groundbreaking studies of elderly twins over the past two decades have shown that both nature (genetics) and nurture (diet and behaviors) contribute to macular degeneration, and her research team and collaborators have identified a majority of the known genes associated with this disease. Her discoveries of modifiable factors for age-related eye diseases include the beneficial effects of the antioxidant nutrients lutein and zeaxanthin, as well as anti-inflammatory foods containing omega-3 fatty acids, and the adverse effects of smoking, obesity, and abdominal adiposity. The author of more than 250 scientific papers, book chapters, and review articles, she has received numerous awards and honors for her pioneering research and contributions to the fields of ophthalmic epidemiology, genetics, nutrition, and macular degeneration.

Contributors

Lidia Matticchio Bastianich is a television chef, best-selling cookbook author, restaurateur, and owner of a food and entertainment business. Her cookbooks include *Lidia Cooks from the Heart of Italy* and *Lidia's Italy*—both companion books to the Emmy-nominated television series *Lidia's Italy*—as well as *Lidia's Family Table, Lidia's Italian-American Kitchen, Lidia's Italian Table,* and *La Cucina di Lidia.* Lidia is the chef/owner of four acclaimed New York City restaurants—Felidia, Becco, Esca, and Del Posto (awarded four stars by *The New York Times*), as well as Lidia's in Pittsburgh and Kansas City. She and her family also own Eataly, the largest artisanal Italian food and wine marketplace in New York City. Lidia has taken her passion for education and enrichment through food, making culinary classes a defining focus of Eataly. As dean of La Scuola at Eataly, Lidia is responsible for the culinary curriculum for the food and wine courses, demonstrations, and lectures from renowned chefs and food and wine producers.

Randi Konikoff Beranbaum, MS, RD, LDN, is a nationally recognized nutritionist and managing editor of *Nutrition Today*. She is also the author of numerous articles appearing in *Tufts Health and Nutrition Letter, Cooks Illustrated Magazine*, and *Glamour*.

Scott Uehlein is corporate chef for **Canyon Ranch**, overseeing the food and beverage programs at all resorts, hotels, SpaClubs, and Living communities. The author of several Canyon Ranch cookbooks, Scott trained at the Culinary Institute of America in Hyde Park, New York, and studied with Madeleine Kamman at her school for American chefs at the Beringer Vineyards in Napa Valley, California. Under Scott's direction, Canyon Ranch cuisine has been given top honors by *Condé Nast Traveler* and *Gourmet* magazines, which stated that chef Uehlein and his staff "have brought Canyon Ranch cuisine into a new dimension." Scott has been highlighted in *Bon Appetit, Self, Fitness, Food Arts, Esquire, Nation's Restaurant News, Chef Magazine,* and *Health & Fitness UK*.

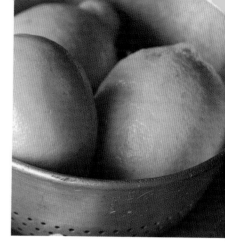

Ina Garten was working in the White House Office of Management and Budget in 1978, eager to do something more creative. She was struck by an ad in *The New York Times* for a specialty food store for sale in the Hamptons, and soon enough, Ina and her husband were driving to Long Island to see the store. Her offer was accepted— and so it began. Barefoot Contessa became a store celebrated both for its style and delicious food. Ina is the author of seven *New York Times* bestselling cookbooks, including *The Barefoot Contessa Cookbook, Barefoot Contessa Parties!, Barefoot Contessa Family Style, Barefoot in Paris, Barefoot Contessa at Home, Barefoot Contessa Back to Basics, How Easy Is That?,* and *Foolproof.*

Green Street Café was for many years one of the best restaurants in Northampton, Massachusetts. The ever-changing menu of French cuisine featured herbs and vegetables from local organic gardens. We thank Jim Dozmati and John Sielski for their recipe for this cookbook, for their pot o' crème, and for their hospitality.

Located in the Texas Hill Country, **Lake Austin Spa Resort** has received awards and been honored by many magazines, including *Condé Nast Traveler, Travel + Leisure, Allure, Health, Garden Design,* and *U.S. News & World Report*. Executive chef Stéphane Beaucamp attended the Belliard culinary school in Paris before apprenticing at the Hôtel Plaza-Athénée, then cooking at several Parisian landmark restaurants. His first experience with health-conscious cookery was at the spa of Enghien-les-Bains, just outside Paris. He became executive chef at the Buddha Bar, working under Kazuto Matsusaka—a pioneer of Asian fusion cooking. This led Beaucamp to Los Angeles, where he first worked at the Bouchon Bistro Lyonnais, then became executive chef and pastry chef at Vermont Restaurant. It was the eco-friendly, organic lifestyle that drew him to Lake Austin Spa Resort.

Jacques Pépin grew up in the kitchen of his family's restaurant near Lyon, France, which led to the young boy's first apprenticeship at age 13 at the Grand Hotel de L'Europe. Pépin later served as personal chef to such French elites as Charles de Gaulle before moving to New York in 1959. The celebrated author of numerous books and host of popular television shows, he received the Chevalier de L'Ordre du Mérite Agricole in 1992, Chevalier de L'Ordre des Arts et des Lettres in 1997, and the French Legion of Honor in 2002. In 2005, he was inducted into the James Beard Cookbook Hall of Fame.

Debra Samuels, who lives in Japan with her family, has taught cooking and written many articles on Japanese food and culture for American and Japanese magazines and newspapers. The American embassy has sponsored Debra's cooking demonstrations throughout Japan. In the United States, she has designed and led cooking programs on *obento*, the popular Japanese lunchbox, for civic groups, universities and for the Japanese embassy in Washington, DC. She is the coauthor with Taekyung Chung of *The Korean Table* and author of *My Japanese Table: A Lifetime of Cooking with Friends and Family*.

Alice Waters, owner of Chez Panisse Restaurant in Berkeley, California, has championed local, sustainable farms for over four decades. She is the founder of the Edible Schoolyard at Berkeley's Martin Luther King Jr. Middle School, a model public education program that integrates edible education into the core curriculum and brings children into a new relationship to food with hands-on planting, harvesting, and cooking. The mission of her nonprofit organization, the Edible Schoolyard Project, is to gather and share the lessons and best practices of school gardens, kitchens, and lunch programs worldwide. Waters is also the author of 10 books, including *40 Years of Chez Panisse: The Power of Gathering, The Art of Simple Food: Notes and Recipes from a Delicious Revolution,* and *The Edible Schoolyard: A Universal Idea*.

Andrew Weil, MD, is director of the Arizona Center for Integrative Medicine at the University of Arizona, pioneers in developing a comprehensive curriculum in integrative medicine. Dr. Weil is also the editorial director of the popular website DrWeil.com, and appears in programs on PBS. He is a founder and co-owner of True Food Kitchen restaurants and an internationally recognized expert and guest speaker on medicinal plants, alternative medicine, and the reform of medical education. Dr. Weil is the author of many scientific articles and of eleven books, including *Eating Well for Optimum Health: The Essential Guide to Food, Diet, and Nutrition,* and *Why Our Health Matters: A Vision of Medicine That Can Transform Our Future*.

Metric Conversion Charts

VEGETABLES AND HERBS		
Barley (cooked)	2 cups	314 g
Basil leaves (chopped)	¼ cup	6 g
Bean sprouts	¾ cup	148 g
Bell pepper (chopped)	1 cup	108 g
Bell pepper (thinly sliced)	1 cup	112 g
Broccoli florets	2 cups	134 g
Green cabbage (shredded)	6 cups	1020 g
Carrots (chopped)	½ cup	122 g
Carrots (julienned)	1 cup	110 g
Carrots (coarsely grated)	2½ cups	265 g
Celery (chopped)	½ cup	122 g
Chives (chopped)	½ cup	24 g
Cilantro (chopped)	⅓ cup	4 g
Cilantro (chopped)	¼ cup	3 g
Corn kernels	1½ cups	328 g
Corn kernels	4 cups	875 g
Cremini mushrooms	1 cup	90 g
Guacamole	2 cups	480 g
Kale (chopped)	1 cup	67 g
Mint leaves (chopped)	½ cup, lightly packed	10 g
Onion (diced)	½ cup	75 g
Parsley (chopped)	¼ cup	5 g
Pumpkin, canned	¾ cup	180 g
Scallions (chopped)	½ cup	50 g
Snow peas	1 cup	98 g
Snow peas (julienned)	1½ cups	147 g
Spinach	1 cup	225 g
Sun-dried tomatoes, packed in oil	¼ cup	28 g
Tomatoes (chopped)	2 cups	400 g
Tomatoes, canned (crushed)	1 cup	244 g
FRUIT		
Blueberries	1 cup	145 g
Dried cranberries	¼ cup	57 g
Currants	¼ cup	28 g
Goji berries (dried)	⅓ cup	43 g
Grapes (halved)	¾ cup	69 g
Pineapple (diced)	1 cup	155 g
Strawberries	1 cup	200 g
Watermelon (cubed)	4 cups	540 g
BEANS AND GRAINS		
Brown rice (cooked)	1⅓ cups	258 g
Buckwheat groats	1 cup	180 g

Cannellini beans (dried)	2 cups	400 g
Edamame (shelled)	1 cup	142 g
Lima beans	2 cups	504 g
Long-grain white rice	½ cup	93 g
Masa harina	¾ cup	87 g
Quinoa (dry)	1 cup	170 g

NUTS AND NUT BUTTERS

Almonds (whole)	2 cups	284 g
Peanut Butter	¼ cup	64 g
Peanuts (chopped)	¼ cup	30 g
Peanuts (chopped)	⅓ cup	40 g
Pecans	¼ cup	30 g
Pistachios (chopped)	½ cup	50 g
Walnuts (finely chopped)	½ cup	65 g

DAIRY

Cheddar cheese (grated)	1 cup	112 g
Goat cheese	¼ cup	28 g
Parmesan cheese (grated)	½ cup	50 g
Greek yogurt	½ cup	114 g
Plain yogurt	1 cup	250 g

BUTTER

¼ cup	½ stick	57 g
½ cup	1 stick	113 g

MISCELLANEOUS PANTRY ITEMS

All-purpose flour	2 cups	240 g
Bottled chestnuts	¾ cup	107 g
Bread crumbs	1 cup	112 g
Brown sugar	½ cup, firmly packed	99 g
Chocolate chips	1½ cups	336 g
Cocoa powder	½ cup	43 g
Coconut flakes	¼ cup	60 g
Confectioners' sugar	⅓ cup	41 g
Ice	½ cup	70 g
Ketchup	¼ cup	60 g
Mayonnaise	¼ cup	52 g
Mellow white miso	¼ cup	64 g
Sour cream	½ cup	96 g
Sugar	½ cup	100 g
Sugar	⅓ cup	66 g
Thai red curry paste	¼ cup	55 g
Udon noodles	3 cups	480 g
Whole wheat pastry flour	2 cups	240 g

WEIGHTS		
3 ounces		85 g
3.75 ounces		106 g
4 ounces	¼ pound	113 g
5 ounces		142 g
6 ounces		170 g
7 ounces		198 g
8 ounces	½ pound	227 g
9 ounces		255 g
10 ounces		283 g
12 ounces		340 g
13.5 ounces		383 g
14 ounces		397 g
15 ounces		425 g
16 ounces	1 pound	454 g
21 ounces		595 g
24 ounces	1½ pounds	680 g
28 ounces		794 g
32 ounces	2 pounds	907 g
48 ounces	3 pounds	1,361 g

TEMPERATURES	
75°F	24°C
80°F	27°C
110°F	43°C
115°F	46°C
145°F	63°C
160°F	71°C
325°F	163°C
350°F	177°C
375°F	191°C
400°F	204°C
425°F	218°C
450°F	232°C

VOLUMES		
4 cups	32 fl oz	950 ml
2 cups	16 fl oz	475 ml
1 cup	8 fl oz	250 ml
¾ cup	6 fl oz	185 ml
½ cup	4 fl oz	125 ml
⅓ cup	2⅔ fl oz	80 ml
¼ cup	2 fl oz	60 ml
2 tablespoons	1 fl oz	30 ml

LENGTHS	
⅛ inch	3 mm
¼ inch	6 mm
½ inch	13 mm
¾ inch	19 mm
1 inch	2.5 cm
2 inches	5 cm
5 inches	13 cm
6 inches	15 cm
8 inches	20 cm
9 inches	23 cm
10 inches	25 cm
12 inches	30 cm
13 inches	33 cm
16 inches	41 cm

Methodology

Eat Right for Your Sight®, the cookbook of the American Macular Degeneration Foundation, applied the ESHA Research's Genesis® R & D database to analyze the nutrition information for all of the recipes. ESHA's database contains information for more than 40,000 foods, food items, raw materials, whole foods, chemicals, the latest USDA data, and other food industry ingredients compiled just for Genesis customers. ESHA Research software is a current and reliable nutritional analysis program and uses the USDA Standard Reference database. ESHA is updated with the latest USDA release every year, and USDA foods make up approximately 25 percent of the data. Additionally, ESHA uses manufacturer data, which make up approximately 53 percent of the database. The ESHA database reports 160 nutrients and nutritional components that are individually sourced. Individual sourcing allows ESHA to keep an accurate, verifiable record of every data point—a key to nutritional accuracy. ESHA provides volume and measures for each food as appropriate. Additionally, for recipe purposes, ESHA provides data that allow users to take into account the

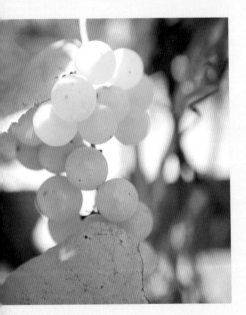

cooking and processing losses that occur during recipe preparation. For the cookbook, each recipe's ingredients were entered into the ESHA databases using the closest match available and analyzed for the following: total energy (kcal)(calories), protein (g), total fat (g), saturated fat (g), fiber (g), vitamin A (IU), vitamin C (mg), vitamin D (IU), vitamin E (IU), sodium (mg), zinc (mg), omega-3 fatty acids (g), beta-carotene (µg), lycopene (µg), and lutein and zeaxanthin (µg). Some of these nutrients have been related to ocular health, specifically macular degeneration. Each recipe uses serving sizes assessed at the time the foods were made. Depending on portion size and cooking variants such as evaporation, the nutrient density may vary.

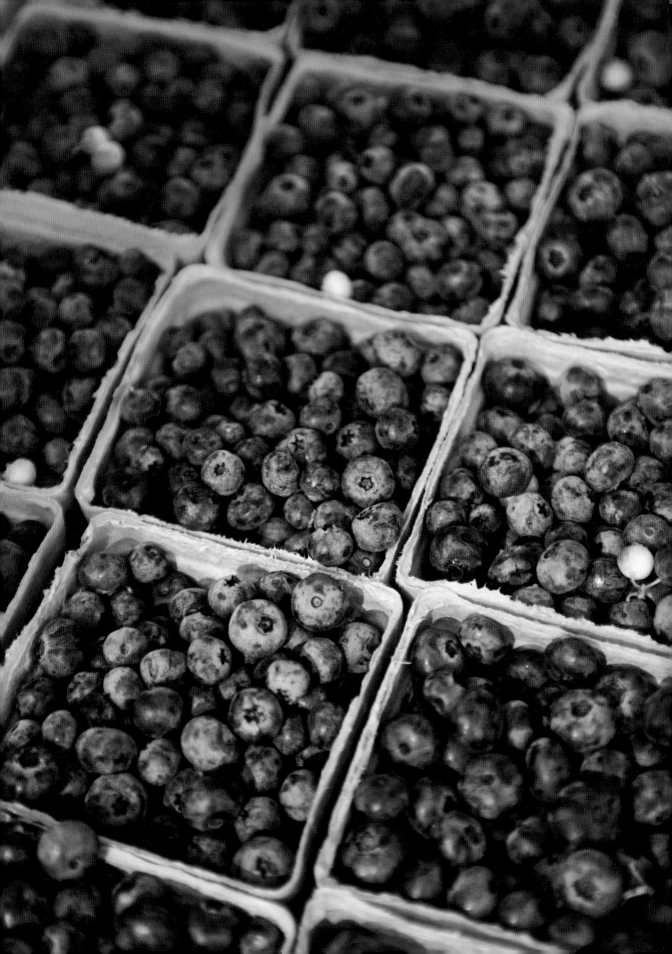

The nutrients were calculated using standard measurements, and all were rounded up if the decimal was higher than 0.5. Rounding nutrient values is one of the steps in formulating nutrition labels. Currently, there are no internationally recognized rounding rules for nutritional information on food labels (i.e., rounding is not specified in the Codex Guidelines on Nutrition Labeling). However, rounding rules can be found in many nutrition labeling regulations/guidelines worldwide. Different rounding rules may be applied on different nutrients and/or different concentrations of the same nutrient.

Acknowledgments

A book of this sort takes a community of talents, and there are many people to thank. This project would not have been possible without the groundbreaking research of Dr. Johanna Seddon, one of America's leading experts in the field of age-related macular degeneration. Seddon, with her staff and collaborators at Tufts University School of Medicine, has conducted seminal nutritional studies of eye diseases over the past 25 years. Thanks to her guidance and research discoveries, this book features ingredients and recipes that are beneficial to eye health. Chip Goehring, president of the American Macular Degeneration Foundation, was also key. He had a concept for the book and set it in motion, always insisting quietly on excellence. What a pleasure to work with Chip—he made it possible to assemble the stellar team of photographer Jason Houston, designer Hans Teensma, manager Rosalind Torrey, food stylist Catrine Kelty, and assistant Jodi Fijal. We also benefited from data from nutritionist Randi Konikoff Beranbaum, MS, RD, LDN, and the following generous recipe contributions:

Page 32: Fish Soup with Vegetables © 2009 Lidia Matticchio Bastianich

Page 52: Miso Soup © 2011 Debra Samuels

Page 58: Tuscan Kale Salad © 2012 Andrew Weil, MD

Page 90: Salmon with Peppered Balsamic Strawberries, courtesy of Canyon Ranch Cooking

Page 94: Grilled Herbed Tuna on Spinach Salad © 1994 Jacques Pépin

Page 109: Rice Paper Salmon with Satay Drizzle, courtesy of Lake Austin Spa Resort

Page 120: Pumpkin Pappardelle, courtesy of Canyon Ranch Cooking

Page 125: Red Curry Vegetables with Coconut Sauce, courtesy of Canyon Ranch Cooking

Page 129: Spicy Udon Noodles © 2003 Lake Austin Spa Resort

Page 131: Jacques Pépin's Provence Pizza © 1994 Jacques Pépin

Page 138: Alice Waters's Cannellini Beans and Wilted Greens © 1996 Alice Waters and the Cooks of Chez Panisse Tango Rose Inc.

Page 140: Ina Garten's Confetti Corn © 2008 Ina Garten

Page 145: Chez Panisse's Spicy Broccoli Vegetable Sauté © 1996 Alice Waters and the Cooks of Chez Panisse Tango Rose Inc.

Page 163: Spa Baklava © 1998 Canyon Ranch Cooking

Lastly, this book is better for the smart input and contributions by Jeanne Besser, Deborah Geering, Trisha Thompson, Virginia Willis, Lisa Ekus, Lynne Bertrand, Paul Rocheleau, Paul F. Gariepy, Karen J. Westergaard, Mark Torrey, and George and Sydney Torrey. A final thanks to Gary Schiff, who introduced me to Chip, and suspected we'd bond over food, oriental rugs, and the Beatles.

—Jennifer Trainer Thompson

Index

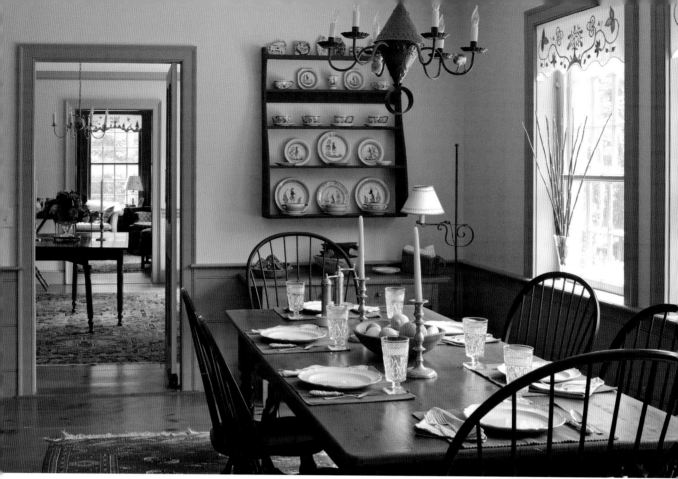

PAUL ROCHELEAU

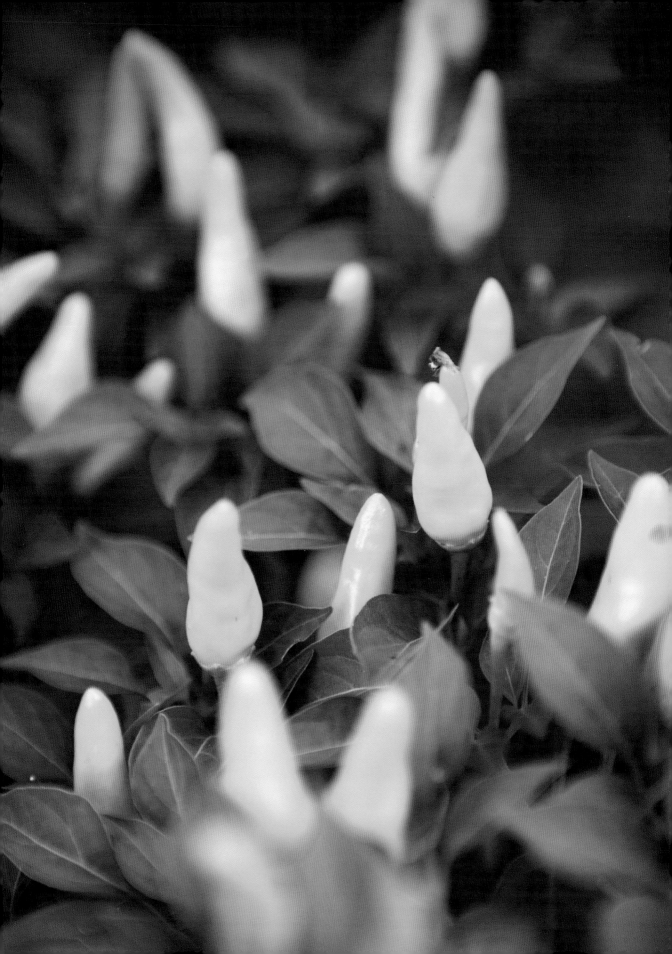

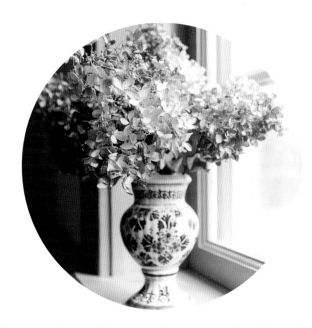

The American Macular Degeneration Foundation
The mission of the American Macular Degeneration Foundation
is to work for the prevention, treatment, and cure of macular
degeneration by raising public awareness and knowledge
about the increasing threat of macular degeneration,
providing support and advocacy for those afflicted
with the disease and their families, and
supporting scientific research.

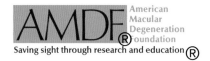

American Macular Degeneration Foundation
P. O. Box 515, Northampton, MA 01061-0515
macular.org   Email: **amdf@macular.org**
Phone: 1.888.MACULAR (622.8527)